SURVIVING WHIPLASH

SAVING YOUR NECK
WITHOUT LOSING YOUR MIND

SURVIVING WHIPLASH

SAVING YOUR NECK
WITHOUT LOSING YOUR MIND

Mark Frobb MD

OrthoWellness Publications

Copyright © 2009
OrthoWellness Publications
All rights reserved, including the right to
reproduce in whole or in part in any form.
ISBN 978-1-4392-0897-7

To order additional copies
and discounted bulk orders

Contact

OrthoWellness Publications
1661-128 ST.,
SURREY, BC, V4A 3V2
CANADA
604-531-9772
Toll Free: 1-877-531 9772
www.OrthoWellnessPublications.com

Library of Congress Cataloguing-in-Publication Data
Library of Congress Control Number: 2008909513

Transcontinental Printing
Printed in Canada

Surviving Whiplash
Saving Your Neck Without Losing Your Mind
Mark Frobb MD

BISAC category
(1) HEALTH & FITNESS / Pain Management

*… If I am not for myself
who will be?*

… Hillel the Elder

CONTENTS

SECTION II: YOUR RECOVERY

SECTION III: YOUR RIGHTS

SECTION IV: REBUILDING YOUR LIFE

SECTION V: ONE-STOP WHIPLASH REFERENCE GUIDE

HOW TO USE THIS BOOK:
WHAT YOU NEED TO KNOW NOW

If you are reading this, chances are you or a loved one are uncomfortable, anxious and looking for answers. You've come to the right place.

Surviving Whiplash: Saving Your Neck Without Losing Your Mind is a comprehensive handbook to help you navigate the pain and frustration of this very illusive and costly injury. The sooner you understand **Your Injury, Your Recovery,** and **Your Rights,** the more satisfactory your outcome is likely to be.

SECTION I.   YOUR INJURY

Chapter 1. The Whiplash Landscape
Chapter 2. What is Whiplash?
Chapter 3. Whiplash-Associated Disorders:
     Signs and Symptoms

This section lays the foundation for your recovery. Your first step is to familiarize yourself with *The Whiplash Landscape*, better enabling you to negotiate the terrain you are about to encounter. This introduction dispels some of the most common myths associated with whiplash and sets your compass for fighting back to physical and financial health.

By understanding the anatomy of your condition you become a more confident champion of your own resolution. No one knows how you feel better than you, not even your healthcare provider. Reading this book arms you with information—the very first step toward ensuring a successful outcome.

SECTION II.   YOUR RECOVERY

Chapter 4. Treating Whiplash-Associated
           Disorders
Chapter 5. How Much Treatment is Enough?

This section details the comprehensive list of tools at your disposal, first and foremost being *your active participation and direction in your recovery*. The goal is to regain the life you had prior to your injury; the specific, multidisciplinary strategies for pursuing this objective are detailed here.

SECTION III.   YOUR RIGHTS

This section answers the multitude of questions you are undoubtedly struggling with now that you have been abruptly thrust into the litigative process. What you don't know can hurt you when dealing with insurance companies and the legal system. Make no mistake, the role of the insurance adjuster is to save the insurance company money.

First, this section gives you the template to comprehensively document your accident and your injury. Next, it delves into the motivations and techniques of the insurance adjuster and the design of the legal system to resolve conflict—helping you better understand the events to come. Finally, it discusses the objective tests available to prove your case. Preparation will help you become the savvy self-advocate you need to be to secure the comprehensive medical and financial support you deserve.

SECTION IV. REBUILDING YOUR LIFE

Eventually the litigative process surrounding your whiplash injury will come to a conclusion. This section motivates you with the good news that awaits and the strategies to ensure ongoing improvement. It provides you with the strength to continue when you feel there is no end in sight.

SECTION V. ONE-STOP WHIPLASH REFERENCE GUIDE

Appendix A. Glossary:

All the terminology you can expect to encounter, along with definitions and explanations of the tests, tools, and treatments for whiplash-associated disorders.

Appendix B.
Documenting Your Accident:

- A checklist to ensure you don't miss the details that will be critical to your treatment and your potential financial settlement.

Documenting Your Treatment:

- A checklist to assist you in charting the course of your recovery—especially useful when accessing a multidisciplinary approach and/or preparing documentation for a potential litigative process.

Appendix C. Care Providers and Credentials:

All the healthcare providers and qualifications you should know about when choosing the healthcare team that will ensure your optimum whiplash recovery.

SECTION I
YOUR INJURY

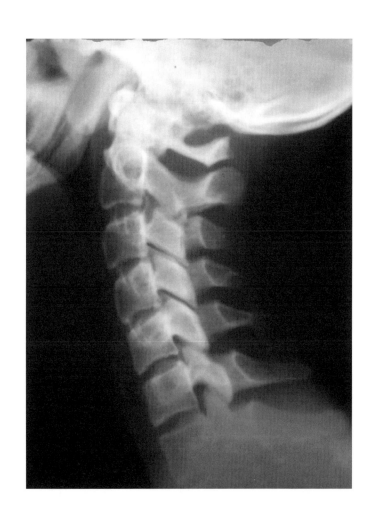

THE WHIPLASH LANDSCAPE: *KNOW THE TERRAIN*

"I'm in pain. I'm worried. Where do I go from here?"

Whiplash is the most common injury resulting from motor vehicle collisions. The good news is, most cases will resolve on their own, without any significant need for care or treatment. For the less fortunate few, the hard fact remains, whiplash-associated disorders (WAD) are a significant cause of chronic disability. Let's begin by dispelling a few of the myths likely to cause you the most grief.

Myth: "If there's no visible damage to the vehicle, there's no chance of whiplash."

Fact: Significant whiplash injuries can occur without any major damage to the victim's vehicle.

Whiplash can occur in any vehicle collision—and at surprisingly slow speeds. Most common causes of whiplash injuries are rear-end collisions. They can, however, occur with T-bone impacts (the front of one vehicle striking the side of the other).

3

THE WHIPLASH LANDSCAPE: *KNOW THE TERRAIN*

The energy transfer during the collision alters the normal curve of the neck, affecting the vertebrae and their supporting soft tissues (including muscles, fascia and ligaments) as well as the spinal nerves.

WHIPLASH INJURY- PHASE 1

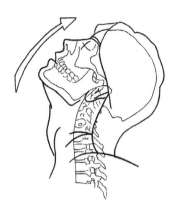

The forces experienced during the collision surpass the tolerances of the soft tissues, causing tearing and shearing of the supporting ligaments and muscles. The hyperextension of the neck causes traumatic compression of the discs between the vertebrae and jamming of the connecting joints (apophyseal facet joints) between the vertebrae. These joints serve to connect each of the cervical vertebra to the ones above and below, and are responsible for the smooth articulating movement of the cervical spine.

Automobile insurance companies have increasingly adopted a "No Crash, No Cash" policy regarding minimal damage to involved vehicles. This hardline approach further contributes to the stress and anxiety of whiplash victims, who are sincerely trying to put their lives back together.

WHIPLASH INJURY- PHASE 2

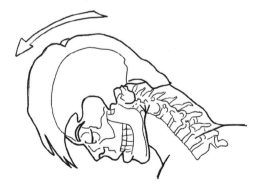

Myth: "The extent of the whiplash injury can easily be determined by the medical examination."

Fact: Clinical examination even by experienced physicians and therapists may fail to clearly identify the extent of the injury or the timeframe necessary for rehabilitation and resolution.

Clinical findings in whiplash-associated disorders normally demonstrate a reduction in range of motion of the neck and upper back as well as localized pain to touch—but these clinical findings seldom provide significant clues to the extent of the injury or the long-term prognosis associated with the injury, *even with appropriate therapy.*

Myth: "If you didn't hit your head, you can't have a concussion."

Fact: In addition to the traumatic injuries to the neck itself, it is possible to cause concussive injuries to the brain even in the absence of striking the head to some part of the vehicle or another occupant. These injuries, known as Mild Traumatic Brain Injuries (MTBI), may be responsible for long-lasting effects resulting in ongoing disability and impairment.

> **MYTH: *"A whiplash injury is a whiplash injury and treatment for whiplash injuries is much the same for everyone."***
>
> **FACT: Treatments for whiplash injuries are marked by idiosyncrasy, meaning that what works for one patient may not necessarily work for the next, even though the symptoms may be identical.**

As mentioned earlier, most whiplash-associated injuries will resolve without the need for intensive therapy. A feeling of stiffness of the upper back and neck that resolves spontaneously over a course of two to three weeks, where the individual does not even feel the need to present for care, is unlikely to run into any future problems.

Significant pain from the onset, however, especially pain that interferes with the activities of daily living, should be addressed immediately. The best window of opportunity for resolving whiplash-associated injury is in the first three months following the accident. Pain that is still present after three months, unfortunately, may still remain at 12 months. Pain at 12 months may very likely be there for years.

This unfavorable prognosis of persistent pain in chronic cases is likely attributable to physiological changes that occur at the site of injury. With the physical disruption of the soft tissues, irritant chemicals leak into the site surrounding the local nerve endings. These noxious chemicals create an "inflammatory soup", which causes sensitization of the local nerve endings, often responsible for the chronic pain conditions that result in long-term disability.

This is not meant to imply hopelessness, for there is likely effective treatment even for these individuals. It is, however, meant to strongly encourage early attendance for treatment. Many stoic individuals may choose to adopt a watch-and-wait approach to seeking care. While this is not unreasonable in mild cases, if symptoms persist after several weeks, therapeutic intervention can become more problematic and the prognosis less positive.

As a spinal care physician who has treated whiplash injuries for over three decades, I would very much like to see patients earlier, even if only to give reassurance, rather than seeing the patient at a later stage when I recognize the treatment program is going to be prolonged, complicated, and decidedly less satisfactory for the patient.

After whiplash patients have been in treatment for some time, they will often identify those treatments that provide the most relief for particular aspects of their injury. Patients should give themselves credit for their ability to recognize which treatments provide the best relief for particular aspects of the injury, and use that knowledge to their best advantage.

It is also important to recognize that certain therapies may have a limited benefit in your specific rehabilitation and that it may be necessary to involve more than one therapy, either in association with another therapy or in succession, to advance your therapeutic progress.

MYTH: *"The insurance adjuster's job is to work toward a fair and equitable resolution."*

FACT: While it is not intended to be critical of insurance companies, it is important for the whiplash victim to realize that the insurance adjuster's responsibility does not necessarily lie with the injured party, but rather to the company's obligation to limit claims. Although I accept this may be an unfair characterization of the insurance industry at large, it is best for the whiplash-injured

party to keep their own best interests at heart, and protect these interests by becoming their own well-informed advocate.

The failure of the insurance company to recommend treatment should not be taken as evidence that your injury is minimal. Taking primary responsibility for your injury by visiting your physician, chiropractor or therapist for evaluation and recommendations for treatment is considered good advice.

Insurance adjusters may reference specific studies indicating that whiplash victims who present early for therapy, and have protracted courses of therapy, are likely to be the most symptomatic one-year post-injury. In review of these same studies, there are also the following observations:

- It is very likely that the most significant injuries will be the first to seek therapy, and very possibly these are the same patients to have ongoing symptoms one-year post-injury because of the severity of their injury.

- Authors of the studies making these observations often have automobile insurance companies as major contributors to their research.

THE EMOTIONAL COSTS OF WHIPLASH

In addition to the medical and socioeconomic costs (billions of dollars annually in North America), whiplash also accounts for immeasurable emotional and psychological costs for the victims and their families. The stress associated with pain, chronic disability and impairment can have a significant effect on an individual's well-being and health status. Considerable adjustments to both work and play are often the result for the whiplash patient and their family.

Not surprisingly, a significant number of whiplash victims may find themselves emotionally compromised, necessitating treatment for anxiety-related illnesses, depression and the more increasingly recognized Post Traumatic Stress Disorder (PTSD).

In the absence of clearly defined medical evidence of their injury, the affected whiplash victim will likely feel considerable dismay given the significant pain they are experiencing. This perplexed feeling may turn to anger and frustration with the insurance adjuster whom, in the absence of significant vehicular damage, may imply the victim is simply magnifying symptoms to boost claims for damages.

Encouraged to "get on with it" by doctors, therapists and even family members, the whiplash victim may feel isolated in their pain and suffering.

FIGHTING BACK

The best advice to the whiplash victim: Educate yourself about your injury.

- Understand the biomechanics of the collision and how the energy transfer to the anatomy of your neck caused the framework of your injury
- Understand the different pain generators associated with this complex condition
- Understand the variety of multidisciplinary treatments available to assist in rehabilitating whiplash-associated disorders
- Understand the motivations and techniques of insurance companies when pursuing compensation for your injuries

Becoming an empowered, equal partner in your rehabilitative care will improve your mental state and the positive resolution of your injury. Ultimately, the whiplash victim can and should be their own best doctor and advocate!

Reading Notes:

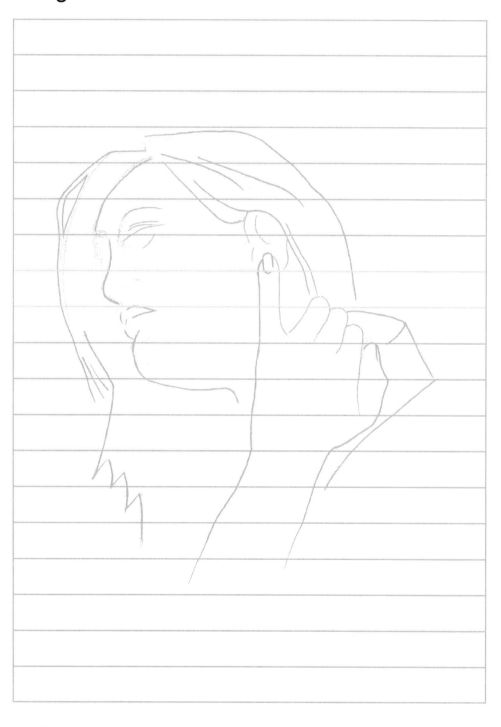

WHAT IS WHIPLASH?

"I've heard the term a million times but what does it really mean?"

Sustaining a whiplash injury is characterized by two separate phases:

Phase 1: forward acceleration of the torso and shoulders with a delayed forward acceleration of the head and neck.

Phase 2: the resulting "whip" of the head and neck as it follows the initial forward movement of the torso and shoulders.

WHIPLASH INJURY- PHASE 1

WHIPLASH INJURY- PHASE 2

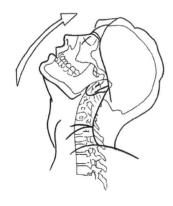

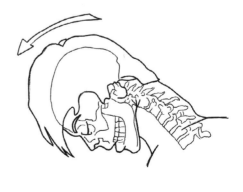

WHAT IS WHIPLASH?

In the first phase, which takes place within the first 100 milliseconds (ms) of the collision, the shoulders and torso of the traveling passengers in the struck vehicle are thrust forward. The head and neck remain relatively stationary at the back of the seat, creating a stretching of the anterior muscles in the front of the neck.

The term "G-force" (G) is a measurement of force or acceleration that the accelerating object "feels". G-forces are caused by changes in speed and direction. On a roller coaster, high positive G-forces are experienced when the car's path curves upwards and riders feel heavy. This G-force is reversed when the car's path curves downwards, creating lower-than-normal G-forces and causing the riders to feel lighter or even weightless.

In the second phase, the head and neck begin their forward journey as they are flung forward in a whip-like phenomenon, after which the injury was originally named. This takes place over the next 200 ms, exactly twice as long as the initial phase. However, the speed of the head's forward propulsion (the stretched front muscles of the neck acting like rubber bands) is significantly faster than the initial movement of the torso and shoulders. In fact, this acceleration phase, whipping the head forward, is magnified by a factor of 2.5x the original collision velocity.

In crash studies documenting this magnification factor, a 6-8 km/h rear-end collision subjects the cervical spine to as much as 4.5 Gs. This is a very important figure, for it is considered by medical specialists to constitute the biological tolerance threshold for cervical spine injury. To place further perspective on these figures, the maximum force allowed on the most violent amusement park rides is 3 Gs.

It has been consistently demonstrated in crash studies, that impacts of 13 km/h or less will consistently produce forces exceeding 10 Gs. A 100-pound female exposed to 10 Gs of dynamic force experiences 800 lbs. of stress to her body. Not surprisingly, energies of this magnitude can produce significant injury to living tissue.

In collisions, these energy-loading forces cause deformation and damage to both the vehicles and the occupants within. Whereas the car damage may result in crumpled or bent metal, shattered plastic and glass, the injuries to the occupants involved translate to damage to the integrity of the discs, nerves, fascia, bones, muscles, tendons, ligaments and joints of the neck.

How Car Design Can Increase Occupant Injury

Modern vehicles are constructed to withstand significant impact before showing evidence of damage. This manufacturing conception has been deliberately implemented to reduce autobody repairs following collision, but the side-effect can be increased occupant injury.

The design factor used in automobile construction is termed *elastic deformation*. In contrast, the design factor used in motorcycle helmet construction is called *plastic deformation*.

In *plastic deformation*, the force of a collision is taken up or dissipated by the helmet. In other words, the helmet shatters on impact, absorbing the force of the collision rather than transmitting the energy to the enclosed head of the wearer.

In *elastic deformation*, however, the vehicle structure remains intact with minimal visible damage at low-impact collisions, but the entire energy force is now transferred to the occupants within the vehicle.

WHAT IS WHIPLASH?

In collision studies, vehicle damage is rarely noted with rear-end impacts involving collision speeds of less than 16 km/h. In fact, vehicles used in as many as 100 to 150 repeated crash tests at speeds as high as 13.5 km/h showed no visible damage—*even though these test speeds register well above the threshold for cervical spine injury.*

It is not surprising therefore, that the amount of damage to the vehicle may bear little relationship to the whiplash-associated injury sustained by the occupants of the vehicle.

The MIST Fallacy

All of these issues have become increasingly more important since the mid-1990s. This decade defined the period when large automobile insurance providers launched a new concept in claims handling called MIST. MIST is an acronym for "Minor Impact Soft Tissue". The theory behind this claim stance was that it was virtually impossible to sustain a permanent or serious injury in a low-damage car crash. This "No Crash, No Cash" policy by insurance companies has resulted in aggressive defensive tactics by defendant attorneys, a policy that continues to be pursued up to the present time.

Many vehicles being built in Europe are now equipped with black boxes installed on the production line. These black boxes, much like the ones on aircraft, measure the collision forces should the vehicle be involved in an accident. With the increasing problems relating to interpretation of forces involved in collision injuries, this production feature may likely be part of the North American production assembly process in the near future.

There are also a number of factors describing the details of the accident that can contribute to increasing peak acceleration of the head and neck in a rear-end collision. Each of the following factors escalate peak acceleration and increase the severity of whiplash injury:

- small struck vehicle
- large striking vehicle
- wet or icy road conditions
- struck vehicle moving at time of impact
- brakes not applied at time of collision
- automatic transmission in struck vehicle

WHY OCCUPANTS CAN SUSTAIN WHIP-LASH INJURY TO DIFFERENT DEGREES

There are factors relating to the occupants of the vehicle that predispose certain individuals to greater injury than might be expected. Some of these are relatively obvious, whereas others may come as a bit of a shock.

Consider that the two phases of whiplash injury take place within 500 ms of the initial collision. This is important because the entire experience occurs before the capability of voluntary muscle contraction. This means that even young healthy individuals are unable to do anything to significantly prepare for the impending consequences of the whiplash injury.

Needless to say, elderly or infirm individuals with weakened muscles, aging neurological systems or arthritic necks do not stand up as well to the forces involved in these collisions and show a greater propensity for injury. Significant arthritis involving the cervical spine may create a situation where the neck becomes much stiffer, behaving under these whiplash conditions more like a "single long bone unit" rather than a composite set of articulating structures.

Women tend to be at a greater risk than men, probably due to lesser muscle mass. Tall individuals with long necks also appear to be at greater risk, possibly from the greater distance of arc that the head must follow creating a more extended range of motion over which the injury can occur.

The position of the head at the time of injury is also significant. If the head is inclined or rotated, such as might occur if looking in the rearview mirror or attending to something on the passenger seat while the vehicle is stopped, there is a greater chance for more significant injury at the time of impact.

It is ironic that seat belts, which are designed for the protection of the occupants of the vehicle, may in fact contribute to increased injury during the whiplash injury. They do so by creating trunk rotation at the time of impact with selective fixation of the shoulder closest to the seat belt attachment on the door frame. They also prevent torso rebound, thereby increasing the flexion moment of maximum acceleration to the cervical spine.

USING YOUR KNOWLEDGE

Many individuals involved in rear-end motor vehicle accidents, who are unaware of the facts that we've just discussed, will necessarily find themselves at a disadvantage. In the absence of any significant damage to their vehicle (as will very likely be pointed out by the insurance adjuster), accident victims might also question whether or not the accident was a main contributor to how they feel—not recognizing that the forces involved in the collision were significant indeed!

Under certain circumstances, it may be necessary to retain specialized consultants to reconstruct the forces involved in whiplash injuries. Accident reconstruction engineers receive graduate-level training in both medical and engineering sciences, and have particular experience in mechanically testing biological tissues. Using photographs of the crash vehicles, repair estimates and bills of repair costs, they are able to provide technical assessments redrafting the collision mechanics. In the course of their analysis, they are able to identify the kinematics of the accident, including the motion of the vehicles, the collision circumstances and the consequent loading of energy of the colliding vehicles. This analysis will provide objective evidence indicating the probability of whiplash-associated disorders.

A good understanding of the biomechanics involved in whiplash-associated injury places the accident victim at a much greater advantage in two capacities. First of all, with their new knowledge, they recognize that the amount of damage to the vehicle may not necessarily indicate the level of injury.

In situations where insurance companies may be unresponsive to the needs of the injured victim, it may be necessary to retain an *Accident Reconstruction Engineer* to convince insurance adjusters and mediators of the underlying collision force dynamics.

Secondly, anticipating the likely stance of the insurance company can be very helpful when faced with an aggressive insurance adjuster. Although it may be necessary to obtain legal counsel in order to receive the necessary funding for treatment and compensation, a firm knowledge base will go a long way to convince an insurance adjuster that the MIST policy they may have adopted does not reflect known scientific evidence, and that you expect the insurance company to facilitate your treatment and rehabilitation to return you to your pre-accident status.

Reading Notes:

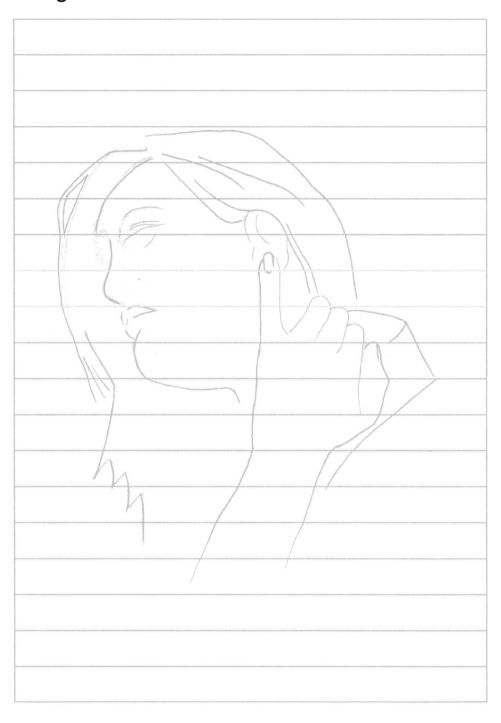

WHIPLASH-ASSOCIATED DISORDERS:
SIGNS AND SYMPTOMS

"This is so much more than a pain in the neck..."

It is not surprising that whiplash patients experience a wide variety of symptoms, considering the diverse anatomical structures of the neck. Further complicating this puzzle are the various degrees of severity of the condition as well as the possibility for a combination of injuries to the area.

GET TO KNOW YOUR NECK

It is useful to think of the neck in terms of its central core (the spinal cord) surrounded by concentric layers that build until you reach the skin. The term "cervical" simply refers to the neck portion of the anatomy.

At the center of the neck, we have the bony skeleton of the cervical spine pro-

CROSS SECTION CERVICAL VERTEBRAE

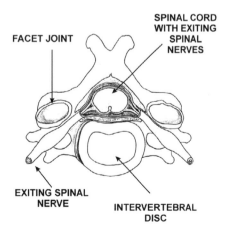

SPINAL CORD WITH EXITING SPINAL NERVES

FACET JOINT

EXITING SPINAL NERVE

INTERVERTEBRAL DISC

tecting its central core, the cervical spinal cord. The cervical spine is made up of seven vertebrae, each of which interconnects with its adjacent neighbors, above and below. The interconnecting joints (apophyseal or facet joints) connecting these vertebral bodies, exist in pairs (2 on the bottom, 2 on the top). They are situated at the posterior aspect (backside) of the vertebrae. It is this complex interlocking system that gives the neck its unique range of motion in an infinite combination of movements.

CERVICAL VERTEBRAE

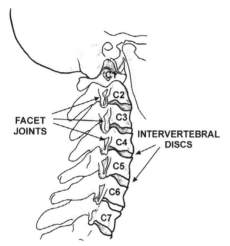

In the discussion of whiplash injury, the facet joints have been implicated as a significant pain generator and for that reason warrant further discussion. In the medical jargon they are referred to by several different terms.

Although these joints are most commonly called the facet joints, they are more properly termed the zygapophyseal joints (abbreviated as Z-joints); a term derived from the Greek roots *zygos*, meaning yoke or bridge, and *physis*, meaning outgrowth. This "bridging of outgrowths" is most easily seen from the lateral or side view, where the Z-joint bridges adjoin the vertebrae. The facet joint is also sometimes referred to as the apophyseal joint or the posterior intervertebral joint.

On the backside at each vertebral body, there is a protective bony arch, through which the spinal cord makes its way from the brain to the lower reaches of the lumbar spine. Between each vertebral body of the cervical spine, the spinal cord gives off a specific cervical spinal nerve which exits through a small opening called a foramen. This foramen is bordered by the interconnecting apophyseal joint. If this joint is affected with degenerative arthritis and further compromised by injury it can result in injury to the spinal nerve, which will produce specific symptoms. Each of these cervical spinal nerves passes to a specific anatomical area of the head, neck, shoulder girdle or arm.

Each spinal nerve is built up of multiple component nerve fibers that provide the sensory function of touch and feel, as well as the detection of pain. They also supply our joints, giving us our sense of proprioception: the ability to know the position of our joints at all times (e.g., whether our hand is opened or closed), even without looking at them.

CROSS SECTION OF NERVE

NERVE SHEATH ENCLOSING NERVE GROUP

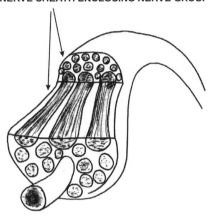

Other nerve fibers within the spinal nerve relate to motor function responsible for enervating muscles, providing strength for movement of the neck, shoulder girdle and upper extremities, and the fine motor coordination of grasp.

ANATOMICAL DRAWING SHOWING
VERTEBRAL BODY IN RELATIONSHIP TO
SPINAL CORD AND EXITING NERVE ROOTS

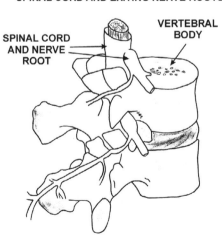

SPINAL CORD
AND NERVE
ROOT

VERTEBRAL
BODY

Between each vertebral body, lies a cushioning intervertebral disc. The outside fibers of the disc are much like the rind of an orange and enclose a jelly-like substance called *nucleus pulposa*. In some whiplash injuries, especially if the disc is already compromised with preexisting degenerative change, the enclosing fibers can rupture allowing the jelly substance to extrude or *herniate*.

CROSS SECTION SHOWING RUPTURED DISC WITH EXTRUDED DISC MATERIAL IMPINGING ON EXITING SPINAL NERVE

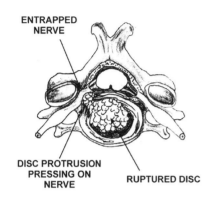

ENTRAPPED NERVE

DISC PROTRUSION PRESSING ON NERVE

RUPTURED DISC

Under these conditions the extruded material (herniated disc) may come in contact with the exiting nerve. This not only causes mechanical irritation by pressing upon the nerve, but chemical irritation with the leaking of irritant fluids that may contribute to inflammation and sensitization of the nerve root.

The next concentric layer of the neck, immediately supporting the skeletal structures, is composed of several layers of ligaments. Some run the entire length of the cervical spine, whereas others run only from one vertebral body to its adjacent neighbor. These layers of ligaments serve to support the spine in its movements, restricting its range of motion to within our physiological limits.

The muscular layer forms the third concentric stratum, but is itself formed of several layers of overlapping muscle. Much like the ligaments, some muscles run longitudinally along the entire length of the spine whereas others are very short and small, and run only from one vertebral body to its adjacent neighbor. Some muscles have the function of fine muscle control for purposes of rotation, whereas others are stronger and more elongated and form the strength muscles of the neck for flexion and extension.

On the outside surface of these muscles we have a

CUT-AWAY SECTION SHOWING CONNECTING LIGAMENTS

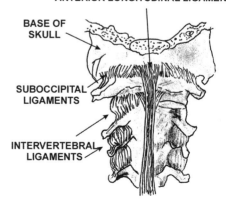

ANTERIOR LONGITUDINAL LIGAMENT

BASE OF SKULL

SUBOCCIPITAL LIGAMENTS

INTERVERTEBRAL LIGAMENTS

strong inter-meshing layer of fascia, which supports the entire muscular system.

Finally, we have the skin with its underlying layer of fat.

A SOUP OF SYMPTOMS

The use of the term "soft tissue injury" refers to an unspecified injury to any or all of the non-skeletal (non-bony) structures that we have just discussed. It also does not differentiate as to whether the injury is minimal or significant in terms of the tearing or shearing forces to which the soft tissues may have been subjected.

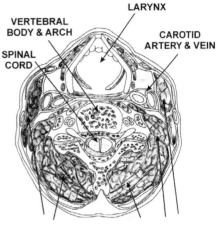

CROSS SECTION OF NECK AT VOICE BOX (LARYNX)

LARYNX

VERTEBRAL BODY & ARCH

CAROTID ARTERY & VEIN

SPINAL CORD

CONCENTRIC LAYERS OF MUSCLES

The presenting complaint that typifies all whiplash-injured patients is pain. Individual patients' descriptions of the pain associated with whiplash may not be identical and are likely indicative of the various combinations of soft tissue or skeletal injuries associated with whiplash-associated disorders. Whereas one patient may interpret their pain as an acute spasm of the associated muscles, other patients will describe a deep-seated pain associated with movement. Still others may report a catching, sharp sensation with specific movements interfering with full range of motion of the spine. As noted, all of these different characteristics of individual pain very likely relate to the various structures that were affected in the whiplash-associated injury.

"I hurt from my head to my hips. That can't all be whiplash, can it?"

Clinical examination may not clearly identify the total injury. Although local tenderness in the superficial muscles may indicate the cause of the superficial pain, other sources of pain generators may be deep within the cervical soft tissues and not so easily identified during the examination process. The spasm in the superficial muscles of the neck may not necessarily reflect local muscle injury, but rather represent a protective splinting phenomenon: an attempt by the body to guard deeper injured structures by restricting movement.

The combination of differing types of pain reflects the complexity of the injury, complicating the initial treatment plan. Because of this, therapy generally progresses in a stepwise fashion, with the attending therapist often pursuing therapeutic management like "layers on an onion".

In other words, what the therapist sees on the initial visit is probably a representation of global inflammation affecting many of the soft tissues, in combination with a protective muscular spasm. Treatment is directed to the anatomical structure most likely causing the pain and the patient is reassessed on the follow-up visit when the next "layer of the onion" can be addressed.

This treatment plan of "examination, treatment, re-assessment" is normally continued throughout the course of rehabilitation with the therapist bringing into play those tools that will most benefit the patient for that specific treatment session.

From this point forward we identify how a particular injury can occur and what types of symptoms it will likely produce.

SKELETAL INJURIES AND FRACTURES

Fortunately, other than in high-speed collisions, major cervical spine fractures with dislocations are rare. In these high-speed collisions, cervical spine fractures may not only cause compression of the spinal cord and exiting nerves but may also be associated with significant vascular injuries to the blood vessels supplying the brain, which may put accident victims at risk for stroke.

RUPTURED INTERSPINOUS LIGAMENT WITH FORWARD SHIFTING OF VERTEBRAL BODY AND COMPRESSION OF SPINAL CORD

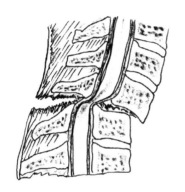

In these high-speed collisions, accident victims are generally subjected to multiple injuries, some which may be immediately life-threatening and preempt all other treatments and investigations until life signs are stabilized.

After attending to those injuries most threatening to loss of life, a detailed examination of the cervical spine will be carried out by the emergency room personnel to address any accompanying spinal injury.

Having said that, there is increasing evidence in the medical literature that micro fractures to the interconnecting apophyseal joints are more common than realized with whiplash accidents. Not visualized with the usual screening x-rays or even the more advanced MRIs, these fractures have been identified at the time of surgical exploration or at postmortem examinations.

"I heard fractures can be missed in x-rays. Is that true?"

When patients present to the emergency department following motor vehicle accidents and whiplash is diagnosed, it is not uncommon for emergency room physicians to order spinal x-rays. The purpose of the spinal x-rays are to rule out obvious compression fractures or dislocations, as failure to recognize these injuries may predispose the accident victim to serious life-threatening complications when not initially identified. This screening tool is especially important in accident victims of elderly age where there may be accompanying osteoporosis (thinning of skeletal bone) and weakening of bony structures.

Even if the radiological exam does not show any evidence of fractures, they will indicate the underlying presence of pre-existing osteoarthritic degenerative changes affecting the intervertebral discs or interconnecting apophyseal joints, identifying those individuals most likely to experience a prolonged convalescence and rehabilitation.

MUSCLE AND LIGAMENT STRAIN SYMPTOMS

Almost all individuals experiencing whiplash will be aware of problems arising from muscle and ligament strain. These symptoms, if

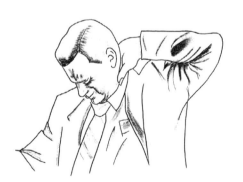

not present immediately, will most likely develop within the first 72 hours following the injury.

The magnitude of the symptom presentation, and the earlier its onset, likely reflects the degree of injury. In some individuals, muscle and ligament strain may be minimal, feeling like little more than a pulled muscle localized to a specific area of the neck.

In others, the symptoms may be more global, involving the entire muscular structure of the shoulder girdle and neck. Symptoms of this magnitude will often be associated with a significant loss of range of motion, with pain elicited with all movements of the head and neck.

It is not uncommon for people who have whiplash disorder also to feel similar symptoms of strain in the low back. The same biomechanical factors that lead to damage of muscles and ligaments in the upper back and neck can equally be applied to the muscles and ligaments in the pelvic girdle and lumbar spine.

Although most people will feel symptoms within the first 72 hours, it is not uncommon for the full spectrum of the whiplash-associated injury to develop over several days. A slight feeling of being shaken up following the accident can sometimes give a false sense of security, the accident victim thinking that they may have "gotten away with this one", only to come to the conclusion over the next several days that they were not so lucky.

On rare occasions, symptoms may not develop for several weeks following the accident. In these circumstances, individuals with whiplash may be initially aware of only marginal stiffness and loss of range of motion of the upper back and neck. In these cases, however, symptoms progress over time, with increasing loss of range of motion and increasing levels of discomfort.

This experience often represents dysfunctional movement at the interconnecting facet joints between the cervical vertebrae. During the whiplash injury, one or more of these facet joints may become jammed, compromising the smooth articulating movement of the cervical spine. As the spine progressively loses range of motion and develops a twisted or torsional position, the supporting spinal muscles develop an increased tension in an effort to pull the spine back into its healthy alignment. This acquired scoliosis (lateral twisting) creates a significant gravitational strain as the muscles work overtime to keep the head erect in the neutral plane alignment, further contributing to the strain of the neck muscles.

The most common pain presentation identified in whiplash-associated disorder involves this muscular and ligament strain of the

MUSCLES IN UPPER BACK AND NECK STRAINED IN WHIPLASH

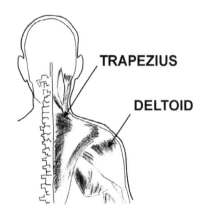

TRAPEZIUS

DELTOID

soft tissue structures of the upper back and neck. This entire injury is generally referred to as a *myofascial pain syndrome*. Myofascial is a Latin derivative with *myo* referring to muscle and *fascial* referring to ligament and fascia.

The muscle and ligament injuries in whiplash may involve muscles both at the front as well as the back of the neck. The front or anterior neck muscles are forcibly stretched during the initial phase of the whiplash arc when the torso and shoulders are thrust forward, while the head and neck remain stationary at the back of the seat.

The most common pattern of muscle and ligament pain associated with whiplash generally involves those muscles and ligaments immediately adjacent to the spine; extending from the very top of the cervical spine at the base of the skull downwards to as far as between the shoulder blades.

The pattern may extend laterally into the muscles across the top of the shoulders and into the muscles between the shoulder blades on each side. It is not uncommon for the pain to also radiate into the upper arms but rarely does the pain radiate further than the elbow, unless there is a significant associated nerve injury.

STRAIN OF FRONT MUSCLES IN PHASE 1 INJURY OF WHIPLASH

STERNOCLEIDOMASTOID MUSCLES

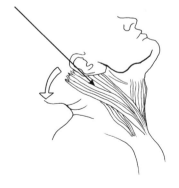

WHIPLASH-ASSOCIATED DISORDERS:SIGNS AND SYMPTOMS

Whiplash patients with significant muscle spasm will frequently experience headache. This specific type of headache, called *cervicogenic* or *muscular contraction headache*, originates from the squeezing and irritation of the exiting spinal nerves by the spastic muscles at the base of the skull. These spinal nerves, called *occipital nerves*, create a distinct pattern of pain when irritated by the constant squeezing of the enclosed spastic muscles.

CLASSICAL SUBOCCIPITAL HEADACHE RADIATING TO FRONTAL AREA ASSOCIATED WITH WHIPLASH INJURY

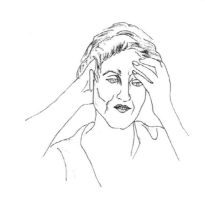

The pain is normally felt emanating from the base of the skull where it travels up across the top and sides of the head to the forehead producing a squeezing sensation around the forehead and temples, giving the affected individual the sensation that they are wearing a hat three sizes too small.

NERVES INVOLVED IN MUSCULAR CONTRACTION (TENSION) HEADACHES IN WHIPLASH INJURY

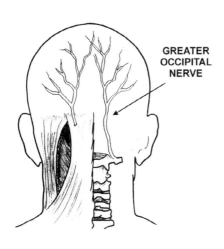

GREATER OCCIPITAL NERVE

All of these myofascial symptoms are likely indicative of small micro tears in the muscles and ligaments supporting the spinal structures. The injury to these muscles and ligaments is caused by the deformation of the spine and supporting tissues during the whiplash injury. The disruption of the normal integrity of the muscles and ligaments results in the leakage of blood, lymph and other irritant fluids into the surrounding tissues, producing an "inflammatory soup" resulting in the painful sensations of warmth or heat, swelling and tenderness.

LIGAMENTS AT BASE OF SKULL

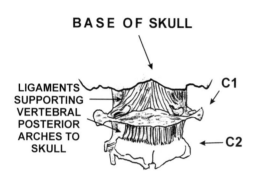

BASE OF SKULL

LIGAMENTS SUPPORTING VERTEBRAL POSTERIOR ARCHES TO SKULL

C1

C2

This inflammatory soup has also been implicated in the prolongation of pain, by sensitizing the nerves at the site of injury as well as the central nerve structures in the brain. Irritation of nerves as they course through an inflamed neck on their way to the arms may also be responsible for some of the pain that radiates into the shoulders and upper arms following whiplash injury.

This acute phase, accompanied by significant pain and stiffness, is by and large associated by a marked loss of range of motion. With the difficulty of turning the head and neck and even the task of keeping the head upright, patients often find the use of a supporting collar helpful to get them through these early days. It is generally not recommended that this supporting neck collar be worn for a prolonged period, as increasing dependence on it will produce atrophy (wasting) of the supporting musculature. In the initial stages, however, it may certainly be called for, if helpful in reducing pain and allowing you to get through your day.

The natural history of this acute phase of the injury in most patients is a gradual resolution over a period of 4 to 6 weeks. In fortunate individuals, the passing of symptoms suggests complete resolution of the injury with an expectation of full recovery to normal status. Many of these patients may not even present for medical care, making the decision to manage the problem on their own with heat or ice packs and over-the-counter muscle relaxants, anti-inflammatories or pain tablets.

Whiplash victims with more significant pain will almost always present for medical attention, either in the emergency department of a hospital, a walk-in clinic or to their family doctor within the first 24 to 48 hours. After evaluation by the attending physician, decisions will be made whether or not to refer the patient for x-rays, CAT scans or MRIs to rule out the presence of fractures or significant disruption of anatomical structures.

Unfortunate individuals experiencing a marked level of discomfort in the initial stages due to the severity of the injury will likely find themselves requiring ongoing medical management and therapy.

NERVE INJURIES

Injuries to nerves are generally felt as pain that radiates into the upper extremities, most commonly past the elbow. This is in contrast to the radiation of pain from injured muscle and ligament discussed earlier, which can also radiate into the arms, but tends to stop in the upper arms and does not travel past the elbow.

Fingers Tell a Story

FRONTAL VIEW OF CERVICAL NERVES

Nerve pain radiating past the elbows will often move to specific finger patterns, assisting the clinician in identifying which specific nerve is involved.

For example, pain and numbness or tingling radiating into the little finger and the adjacent portion of the ring finger is indicative of entrapment or

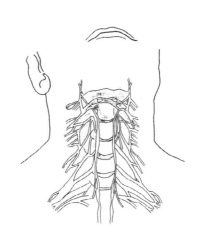

irritation of the 8th cervical nerve, which is the nerve that comes out between the vertebral bodies that form the junction between the lower neck and upper shoulder.

The same symptoms felt in the thumb and index finger are indicative of entrapment of the 6th cervical nerve, which exits from the mid-neck area.

Nerve Structure

The amount of compromise or injury to the nerve is reflected in the symptoms and signs produced. The anatomical structure of a spinal nerve is much like the coaxial cable that connects our televisions to the cable source. Each individual spinal nerve is composed of hundreds of smaller individual nerves enclosed within a sleeve called a neural sheath.

CROSS SECTION OF NERVE

NERVE SHEATH ENCLOSING NERVE GROUP

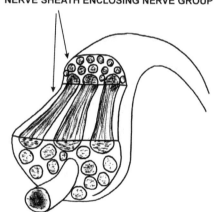

The outside fibers of the spinal nerve are the sensory fibers which allow us to detect touch and feeling, sensations of pain, and are responsible for the sensation of proprioception discussed earlier. Injury or mechanical pressure inflicted on these nerve fibers produces sensations of numbness or paresthesia (tingling, prickling, or burning) along the course of the nerve.

The innermost nerve fibers within the central part of the spinal nerve represent the motor function component of the nerve and comprise the nerve fibers that carry the motor impulses to the muscles, producing contractions, strength, or in the case of hands, the fine motor control represented in the manipulative ability of grasp.

Therefore, if there is only slight irritation or mechanical compression of the spinal nerve, only sensory symptoms are likely to be experienced, as the inner core of the nerve is unaffected. Under these circumstances, the patient is likely to feel numbness or tingling along the distribution of the nerve, but will retain full motor control of the muscles that particular nerve innervates.

Under circumstances where motor control is affected by a demonstrable lessening of strength, clinicians will interpret this as significant pressure being placed on the inner motor fibers of the nerve. This generally means that, the nerve has been anatomically displaced or compressed by damaged or disrupted adjacent structures.

Compromised motor fiber function is demonstrated by a reduction in strength of the affected arm when compared to the unaffected arm in clinical tests. There may also be a decrease in the muscular reflexes of the affected arm when tested with a rubber percussion hammer. In later stages, there will be an obvious loss of muscle mass (atrophy) gauged by measuring the circumference of the arm over time.

Where there are strength deficiencies, it is generally representative of a more severe injury and may be indicative of a prolonged period of convalescence and rehabilitation. Although not common, in some circumstances, there may be need for surgical intervention and decompression to preserve nerve and muscle function.

Causes

Nerve symptoms can result from two different causes. The first is more benign and represents spasm of the muscles around the exiting nerve as it passes through the neck on its way to the upper arm. With relief of the muscle spasm, the nerve function completely recovers without any permanent consequences. Under these conditions, it is less likely for any motor loss to be demonstrated and the findings generally pertain to only the symptoms of sensation, namely tingling or numbness or pain referral to the shoulder and arm.

The second circumstance producing nerve symptoms is more significant and generally will be associated with muscle weakness innervated by a specific nerve. This is less likely to be due to spasm of the muscles in the neck, and generally indicative that the nerve is being pinched within the bony canal (foramen) through which it leaves the spinal skeleton.

A likely cause may be rupture of the disc between the vertebral bodies, which presses upon and displaces the nerve as it exits the spinal canal. It may also be secondary to superimposed injury to pre-existing degenerative osteoarthritis of the apophyseal joints, whereby the canal has been narrowed by secondary bony overgrowth and, with the increased edema (swelling), the nerve root has been sufficiently compromised to produce these symptoms and signs.

In the immediate post-injury phase, there is no need for immediate medical or surgical intervention, as it is the general rule of thumb to watch these injuries for several weeks to see what changes occur in the function of the nerve. Failure to show improvement after this initial observation period, however, may prompt additional investigation including specialized radiological studies or nerve conduction tests to confirm clinical suspicions. Following these investigations, the necessary subsequent care will be determined.

MILD TRAUMATIC BRAIN INJURY (MTBI)

FRONTAL BRAIN COMPRESSED IN PHASE 1 OF WHIPLASH INJURY

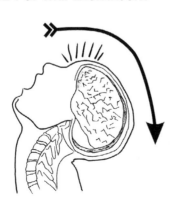

The primary injury of Mild Traumatic Brain Injury (MTBI) is attributed to the movement of the brain within the skull and its resulting collision with its boney encasement. These collisions are referred to as "coup and contrecoup" brain injuries. The end result is traumatic shearing injury to the nerve tissue of the brain leading to swelling and microscopic bleeding.

Symptoms associated with MTBI can often be attributed to other aspects of the injury or even the anxiety associated with the accident: headache, dizziness, concentration difficulties, memory disturbances and other neuropsychiatric and cognitive difficulties.

MTBI is quite possibly under-diagnosed in whiplash-associated injuries. It has become increasingly apparent that traumatic brain injury can occur as a consequence of the acceleration/deceleration forces associated with whiplash, and that this injury can occur *even in circumstances where there is an absence of direct trauma to the head, or explicit loss of consciousness.*

OCCIPITAL BRAIN COMPRESSED IN PHASE 2 OF WHIPLASH INJURY

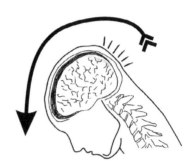

Recovery from this injury is generally marked by sequential improvement over time but persistent symptoms after 12 to 18 months are commonly accepted to represent permanent damage and very probably result in chronic disability and impairment.

POST TRAUMATIC STRESS DISORDER (PTSD)

Being involved in a motor vehicle accident can be a significantly stressful event and, to many people, may represent the only violent assault upon their body experienced in their lifetime.

Some studies report that up to 23% of traffic accident victims may develop Post Traumatic Stress Disorder (PTSD). It is also notable that occupants experiencing whiplash are reported to be more susceptible to this disorder when compared to other crash victims.

Although sharing many of the symptoms associated with MTBI, psychiatric evaluation reveals PTSD sufferers experience higher levels of anxiety, a tendency towards catastrophic interpretation, negative mood swings and magnified pain intensity, findings not generally experienced in crash victims with MTBI.

A significant portion of those diagnosed with PTSD will be appreciably compromised in terms of their ability to return to their accustomed work and possibly even coping with the normal activities of daily living.

It is very likely that these patients will benefit from early referral to psychological counseling and psychiatric treatment, for professional intervention is likely to result in the best clinical outcomes.

CHRONIC PAIN DISORDERS

A significant percentage of whiplash patients will report chronic pain syndromes that persist months to years after their injury. Many may have been in low-velocity collisions, with only minimal damage to the vehicles involved.

These patients find themselves in difficult positions because unlike many other medical conditions for which blood tests can prove underlying disease (e.g., diabetes or rheumatoid arthritis), a whiplash victim suffering from chronic unresolved pain disorders will have little objective evidence to verify the chronic disability they are facing.

Standard medical tests including x-rays, CAT scans and MRIs tend not to be helpful in these circumstances as they are unlikely to confirm the magnitude of the injury. Although they may identify evidence of underlying degenerative changes, these radiological findings likely exist in the normal population of individuals in their age group.

The presence of osteoarthritic degenerative spinal changes is a normal finding in people as they get into the 4th and 5th decade, reflecting the natural aging process, and a significant number of these individuals will have no symptoms whatsoever.

Symptoms of MTBI, PTSD and/or Chronic Pain Syndrome

- *headaches*
- *loss of coordination*
- *reduced drive / motivation*
- *memory difficulties*
- *difficulty finishing tasks*
- *sleep disorders*
- *abnormal levels of anxiety*
- *reduced tolerance to alcohol*
- *increased assertiveness*
- *forgetfulness*
- *angry outbursts*
- *depression*
- *fatigue*
- *absence of ability to anticipate*
- *inflexibility*
- *impaired sexual function*
- *language difficulty*
- *impaired judgment*
- *increasing need for written schedules*
- *increasing need for reminders*
- *blurry vision*
- *loss of balance*
- *difficulty with multitasking*
- *dizziness / lightheadedness*
- *irritability*
- *personality change*
- *hand tremors*
- *ringing in the ears*
- *decreasing diplomacy*
- *mood swings*
- *reduced attention span*
- *blackouts*
- *indifference to people and/or typical interests*
- *more shallow relationships*
- *difficulty with solving problems*

Other specialized brain imaging studies including PET scans, SPECT scans and functional MRIs (*f*MRI) may demonstrate evidence of abnormality, including the existence of disabling pain, but these investigative tools tend to exist only in academic settings and are not readily available for the investigative purposes of demonstrating the presence of chronic pain.

These studies are also not typically ordered by treating clinicians because they do not change the course of medical management. The treatment for whiplash-associated injuries, for the most part, is addressed to the clinical symptoms and physicians are inclined to order tests only if there is significant evidence that additional or different treatment is indicated.

These specialized tests, if ordered, are more likely to be ordered at a later date at the request of legal counsel to provide medical legal evidence to corroborate insurance claims, issues not foremost in the physician's original treatment plan, which is primarily to organize and manage rehabilitation.

SECTION II
YOUR RECOVERY

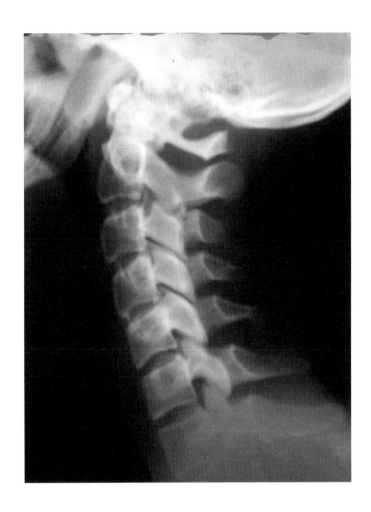

TREATING
WHIPLASH-ASSOCIATED DISORDERS

"Keep still? Keep active? Heat? Ice? Surgery? Massage?
How do I know what's right for me?"

Given the complex anatomy of the neck and the possibility that more than one structure can be injured during the whiplash incident, it is not surprising to know that there are many different modalities of therapy employed in the treatment of whiplash-associated disorder.

In review of the published medical literature, there is a general consensus that no one specific therapy is more beneficial than any other when it comes to treating whiplash. This observation very likely reflects the idiosyncratic nature of individuals' response to soft tissue injuries. It may also indicate that most of these therapies are individually applied with a hands-on technique, and that individual therapists vary in experience and learned techniques.

For this reason, if the patient is not demonstrating measurable improvement using one therapy, it is not unreasonable to try an alternate therapy to see if a better response can be gained—or possibly an alternate therapist.

It is also not uncommon to combine different therapies. An example of such a combination would include combining massage therapy to treat the soft tissue inflammation, with chiropractic treatments being used to treat the dysfunctional movement pattern affecting the underlying vertebral segments.

TREATMENTS IN
WHIPLASH ASSOCIATED INJURY

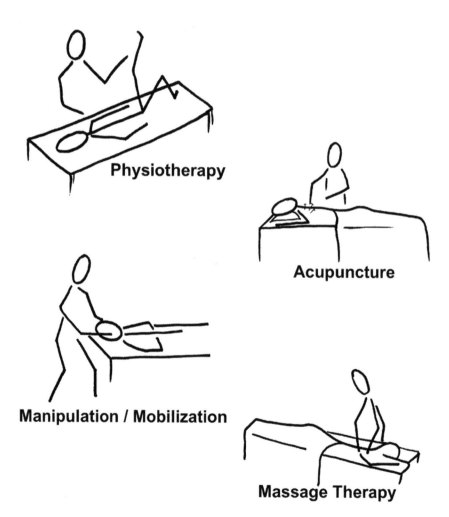

Physiotherapy

Acupuncture

Manipulation / Mobilization

Massage Therapy

TREATING WHIPLASH-ASSOCIATED DISORDERS

This approach to rehabilitative management is quite acceptable as long as the managing therapist is clear in their goals. As much as possible, however, it is almost always best to isolate therapies from one another; if the patient begins to either show improvement or decline in level of comfort, it is difficult to establish which therapy was responsible for which affect. In cases where a patient shows deterioration, the treatment regimen will need to be reassessed and each of the therapies will need to be reinitiated individually, to determine specific cause and effect.

In all cases of rehabilitation in whiplash-associated injuries, there are two major goals. The first is to reduce the level of pain and restore the range of motion and function of the upper back and neck. The second is to re-establish the normal core strength of the supporting musculature of the shoulder girdle and neck structures and restore normal posture.

In reducing the level of pain, it is important to keep in mind the various possible pain generators in whiplash injuries that may be responsible. From the previous chapter, we recall that all of the following injuries may be pain generators and may therefore require individual management strategies.

- micro-tears in supporting musculature with edema and inflammation
- micro-tears in supporting spinal ligaments
- micro-tears in capsular ligaments supporting the interconnecting apophyseal joints
- micro-tears in intervertebral discs
- inflammation in the apophyseal joints secondary to trauma and jamming
- compression or stretching of the exiting spinal nerves

Not all treatments will necessarily address the complete spectrum of the injury. In the earliest phases of the injury, it may not be possible to introduce any physical therapies because a patient's pain tolerance and discomfort with manipulation of the soft tissues may preclude any intervention.

In these earliest phases of treatment, medical management may entail only the use of analgesics or pain killers to moderate the pain, while time allows for the body to begin healing and settle the acute inflammatory changes. The application of heat and ice at this time may be the best available tolerated treatment. Use of a cervical collar may also be helpful in this early stage to assist holding the head upright, reducing the workload of the inflamed supporting muscles.

"I have areas that are excruciatingly painful to touch, but there is no bruising. What's causing this terrible sensitivity?"

As the initial inflammation settles, the doctor or therapist can carry out a more detailed assessment, examining the patient's neck with a complete range-of-motion analysis. This examination will identify those anatomical structures most likely responsible for the production of the current level of pain, facilitating planning of a beneficial treatment program.

Therapeutic management after the acute inflammatory pattern has settled will tend to address the most pressing cause of pain, moving the treatment plan forward in a stepwise fashion. All of this treatment is in pursuit of the patient becoming comfortable enough to address core strength and posture restoration issues and the introduction of the necessary exercise programming.

MYOFASCIAL PAIN SYNDROMES

Myofascial pain syndrome is the term used to describe the generalized soft tissue damage that follows the acceleration/deceleration injury associated with whiplash. These syndromes are characterized by *regional muscular pain patterns*, typically involving a group of muscles responsible for complex movements in a specific area of the body.

Standard Physical Therapies
• ice
• heat
• massage
• ultrasound
• electrotherapy
• shortwave diathermy
• TENS (transcutaneous electrical nerve stimulation)

A typical regional example of a myofascial pain syndrome due to whiplash, would be the shoulder girdle and neck where pain, stiffness and muscle spasm may be noted. The pain patterns may not only be felt locally, but may be accompanied by referral pain resulting in headaches or pain radiating to the upper shoulders and arms.

Trigger Points

Clinical examination of the whiplash patient typically reveals a loss in range of motion of the upper back and neck and evidence of trigger points in the bellies of the individual muscles involved in the pain syndrome.

Trigger points have several characteristics which define their presence, including a taut band or rope-like consistency causing exquisite pain on squeezing; the pain often radiating far from the trigger point itself. Evidence of local nervous system abnormalities may also exist, including skin hypersensitivity to touch, temperature changes on the skin and changes in local blood flow.

TRIGGER POINTS IN WHIPLASH WHICH PRODUCE HEADACHE PATTERNS

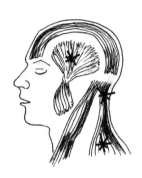

Documented existence of the presence and treatment of trigger points dates back to the 1930s. Medical experts agree that trigger points are characterized by dysfunctional changes in histopathology (microscopic cellular abnormalities), biochemistry, biomechanics, and electrophysiology (nerve cell electrical processing ability). However, in spite of the burgeoning research on myofascial pain syndromes, their exact etiology (source or cause) remains controversial. Although not clearly established at this time, it is likely that future research will reveal a complex interplay between peripheral and central nervous pathways secondary to the soft tissue damage associated with whiplash-associated injury.

Treatments

Many different therapies have been recommended in the treatment of myofascial pain syndromes including the standard physical therapies used by physiotherapists and massage therapists.

Acupuncture, dry needling, and injection therapies both with local anesthetics and saline have also shown to be effective treatments. Botox (botulinium toxin) has also been used in injection therapies with some success. Stress reduction and biofeedback may also be helpful as adjunctive therapies in improving response to treatment.

As noted earlier, the response to treatment of myofascial pain syndromes is marked by an idiosyncratic pattern, meaning that the treatment which works for one person may not produce similar effects in another. Further, what is initially beneficial in one person may not produce the same results over time. If effectiveness becomes static, it may be necessary to attempt other therapies to see if further response is noted.

Unfortunately, maximum medical improvement of the myofascial pain syndrome can be reached without complete resolution of the discomfort. At this point, further improvement can only be expected with time, irrespective of any specific therapeutic intervention.

There are many different disciplines that address the treatment of myofascial pain syndromes. Probably the most time-honored group of professionals focusing on the problems of myofascial pain syndromes are massage therapists.

The "Rule of 6"

- A trial of 6 therapeutic sessions should produce a measurable effect. If there is no progress following 6 visits, there is unlikely to be significant further progress at 12 visits using that particular therapy.

- This does not mean that the problem will have resolved within 6 visits, but there must be a measurable improvement from the initial starting point.

There are many different types of massage therapy used in treatment of myofascial pain syndromes. What is important, regardless of the type of massage, is that both patient and therapist are unhurried in the initial phases of the treatment program, while the therapist learns the tolerances of the patient's soft tissues. Attempts at trying to rush the therapy or do too much in any given treatment session, will often result in an exacerbation and flare-up of symptoms, setting back the whole process.

Most soft tissue therapies will have a ceiling of therapeutic benefit, meaning that the patient will show initial gains but progress will likely level off and eventually stagnate.

MANUAL THERAPIES

Manual therapy is a generic term referring to those therapeutic modalities that fall under the umbrella of mobilization and manipulation. There are several types of professional therapists who practice manual therapy. Very likely the largest group specializing in this type of therapy are chiropractors. Osteopathic physicians also train extensively in manual therapy as do some physiotherapists, massage therapists and kinesiologists.

The "Rule of 3"

- After initial improvement, if 3 treatments go by without further significant improvement, the particular therapy is unlikely to produce further benefits.

- At this point, it is probably best to seek an alternative soft tissue therapy in the pursuit of further progress.

The different types of therapies that comprise manual therapy are diverse and widespread. Whereas many individuals are familiar with the high velocity / low amplitude techniques used by chiropractors, other techniques are also equally efficacious, including, amongst others, muscle energy techniques such as the McKenzie therapies, activator and functional techniques.

The choice of the therapy used by individual therapists relates both to their level of confidence in their application of the therapy, as well as the therapist's experience with positive soft-tissue response to its use.

Manual therapy is indicated when dysfunctional movement is diagnosed after examination of range of motion of the neck. As noted earlier, neck movements occur through the interconnecting apophyseal joints between vertebrae. Each vertebral body contributes to one half of four interconnecting apophyseal joints—2 on the top and two on the bottom, as can be seen in the accompanying drawing.

When all of these interconnecting joints are moving freely, we enjoy a complex range of motion of the neck, allowing lateral rotation as used during shoulder checking in traffic, both left and right, upward gaze and forward flexion—all with freedom of movement and absence of discomfort.

LIGAMENT STRUCTURES SUPPORTING VERTEBRAL BODIES

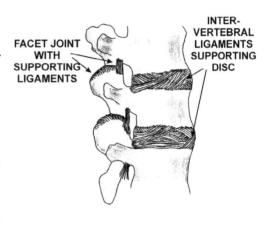

FACET JOINT WITH SUPPORTING LIGAMENTS

INTER-VERTEBRAL LIGAMENTS SUPPORTING DISC

During the mechanism of the whiplash injury, as the cervical spine is hyper-extended, these facet joints are jammed and traumatized by the kinematic forces imposed upon them during the collision. These joints have been clearly identified as one of the main pain generators following whiplash injuries.

During the course of the clinical examination, experienced therapists are able to detect if one of these joints is jammed and blocked in its position, incapable of gliding through its full range of motion. This fixation will result in the spine no longer being in its neutral plane of alignment, and is often referred to by chiropractors as a subluxation.

Increased tension and soreness in the muscles supporting the neck will accompany the malalignment. This spastic muscle pattern occurs as a result of the body's attempt to pull the misaligned vertebral body back into its neutral plane position. The increased fatigue in these muscles, overworking in an attempt to keep the head in an upright position in the presence of the misaligned cervical spine, also contributes to the soreness in the muscle structures recognized in myofascial pain syndromes.

Having recognized the cervical malalignment as being a significant contributor to the existing neck pain, the manual therapist will schedule a series of treatments to gently correct the diagnosed malalignment, which should contribute to further improvement in level of comfort and range of motion.

Much as in the case of the massage therapist, both the patient and the therapist will have to exercise a level of patience, as any attempt to reintroduce the full range of motion too quickly, is likely to create an exacerbation or flare-up of the initial symptoms and underlying myofascial pain syndrome.

An experienced manual therapist will quickly learn the tolerances of the tissues and, within these guidelines, effect a gradual progressive improvement, rather than unsteady progress reflecting cycles of exacerbation and remission.

The same *Rule of 6* referred to in myofascial pain treatments will generally apply to manual therapy treatments as well. If any symptomatic improvement is likely to be noted with manual therapy, it should be detectable after 6 visits. If there is no significant improvement after 6 visits, the patient is unlikely to find further significant improvement at 12 visits. Again, this is not to say that the problem will be resolved at 6 visits, but there should be a measurable improvement to justify continuing therapy.

Treatment should be continued at regular intervals until progress has been stabilized. At that point, the therapist will normally attempt to increase the distance between visits, weaning the patient from treatment, with the expectation that the patient will maintain their level of comfort. It is very likely that exercise programming can now begin in earnest to restore the core strength and re-establish the normal shoulder girdle and neck posture.

MEDICAL MANAGEMENT

It is common to combine the aforementioned physical therapies with traditional medical management. Physicians often prescribe analgesics (pain killers), muscle relaxants and anti-inflammatories during the initial phase of inflammation, to assist patients in getting through this most painful stage of injury.

Although patients are grateful for the pain relief, these specific agents are not without their side effects. Muscle relaxants and pain killers are often accompanied by fatigue and sleepiness and, in the case of narcotics, some alteration in mental focus and concentration. In most cases these drugs should be seen as a brief respite in the initial stages of treatment only, and are generally not recommended for long-term management.

It may be necessary to use anti-inflammatories on a more prolonged basis to address inflammation in the affected joints, especially if there was any pre-existing degeneration due to osteoarthritis prior to the accident.

Anti-inflammatories as well have substantial side effects, the most notable being gastrointestinal irritation. Caution should be exercised in those individuals at risk for ulcers, as this group of drugs is responsible for a significant incidence of gastrointestinal bleeding and hemorrhage requiring hospitalization and resulting in serious medical consequences.

Analgesics, muscle relaxants and anti-inflammatories comprise the most commonly prescribed drugs, especially in the first six weeks following injury. If problems fail to resolve within the first three months, patients may develop chronic pain syndromes which may require additional pharmaceutical management.

As discussed previously, chronic pain syndromes are thought to result from physiological and histopathological changes (microscopic changes in injured or diseased tissue) in the local nerves affected by whiplash. Although the pathophysiology (the disturbance of function that a disease or injury causes in tissue) of chronic pain syndromes has not been clearly explained, one of the more significant contributing factors is thought to be the effect of the irritant chemicals—*the inflammatory soup*—produced by the inflamed and disrupted soft tissue. These nerve pain syndromes, called neuropathic pain syndromes, can be very stubborn in their response to the various therapies, often requiring complex and extensive medical management.

> Neuropathic pain syndromes are not predictably responsive to any specific drug management regime, often making it necessary to try a number of different medications to determine which drug will work best with each patient.

Another of the most commonly prescribed drugs for whiplash injuries are antidepressants, but not for their effect on depression. A side effect of the medication, which is evident even at very small dosages of the drug (1/10th of the dosage prescribed for depression) is relaxation of the muscles involved in the pain syndrome and an overall improvement in the pain syndrome. They also improve sleep patterns resulting in a reduction of fatigue, which may also contribute to improvement in pain patterns.

Other drugs used in neuropathic pain syndromes include the specialized drugs developed for the treatment of epilepsy, called anticonvulsants. When effective they can be a useful adjuvant in the management of chronic pain syndromes, although they may be poorly tolerated by many patients.

SPECIALIZED TREATMENTS

Patients who develop chronic pain syndromes after whiplash-associated injuries, which are unresponsive to the usual therapies, are frequently referred to specialized pain clinics for evaluation and further investigation.

These chronic pain clinics are generally staffed with specialist physicians who may include anesthesiologists, interventional pain physicians, neuroradiologists and other appropriately trained pain specialists.

Through the use of selective anesthetic blocks, attempts are made to identify the specific pain generators responsible for producing the disabling pain associated with chronic unresolved whiplash syndromes.

As discussed earlier, one of the most notable causes of unremitting pain in chronic whiplash syndromes is the apophyseal facet joint. Having identified a specific facet joint as being responsible for the symptoms produced, the joint can be infiltrated with steroids or treated with PRFN (percutaneous radio-frequency neurotomy) to the nerve that supplies the facet joint, thereby moderating the pain level.

Other types of anti-inflammatory injection therapies using a combination of anesthetics and steroids may include epidural injections or selective spinal nerve root blocks to address nerve root irritation.

EXERCISE PROGRAMMING

Exercise is critical to successful management of whiplash-associated injury, particularly attention to recovery of core strength and proper posture of the shoulder girdle and cervical spine.

TREATING WHIPLASH-ASSOCIATED DISORDERS

Within several weeks of an unresolved whiplash-associated injury, there is an increasing pattern of muscle disuse as the individual adapts to the pain by restricting range of motion. This adaptive pattern unfortunately results in an onset of atrophy (muscle wasting) of the involved muscles, fulfilling the old axiom "use it or lose it". Accompanying this muscle wasting, the shoulder girdle and neck begin to deteriorate in postural positioning, as the weakened muscles fail to hold the spine in an upright neutral plane alignment.

> Ultimately, attention to an exercise program completes the rehabilitation process. There is no amount of passive therapy—*regardless of the skill of the therapist*—that will result in resolution of chronic whiplash-associated injury. Diligent attention to exercise programming on a regular daily basis is critical for recovery.

The newly adopted posture is often referred to as the "sniff position", where the head and neck are thrust forward, as one might see in an individual moving about the kitchen searching for the source of a bad odour. This postural position, while adopted to relieve pain, actually compounds the problem by increasing the strain in the supporting musculature across the top of the shoulders.

Over time, the weakened muscles fail to hold the upper thoracic spine in neutral plane alignment. With the weakened core muscles in the upper back, the stronger muscles in the

COMPENSATORY SHIFTING OF POSTURE SHOWING FORWARD MALALIGNED "SNIFF" POSITION

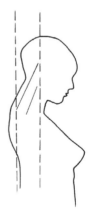

dominant arm and shoulder pull the spine in that direction creating a convex curvature of the upper back towards the direction of the stronger shoulder.

With the rotation of the upper thoracic spine (most commonly to the right in right-handed individuals), the cervical spine above it now rotates in the opposite direction to compensate and keep the head in the midline position. This S-shaped spinal alignment accommodation is referred to as an *acquired scoliosis*.

With this new spinal misalignment, all the muscles in the upper back and neck are now working overtime to keep the head and neck upright against the forces of gravity. This muscle overuse further contributes to the fatigue and inflammation experienced in the supporting muscles and ligaments, becoming a significant contributor to the myofascial pain syndrome, which generally accompanies all whiplash-associated disorders.

The exercise program, in its initial stages, may be little more than a gentle stretching program to begin lengthening the shortened muscles on the concave side of the S-shaped spinal deformations (typically the left side if you are right-handed). As the muscles become more supple with stretching, a progres-

The "10% Rule"

- Establish your baseline: begin at a level of exercise and stretching you know creates no level of discomfort.

- Increase the level of exercise either in repetitions or effort (but not by both) by no more than 10% every 3rd work session.

- Following this rule will result in a gradual, sustained improvement without producing any flare-ups.

sive strengthening program to address the weakness pattern of the muscles can begin. The muscles generally affected with this weakness pattern involve the muscles between the shoulder blades, the muscles at the top of the shoulders as they extend into the upper arms, and the small intrinsic muscles in the upper back and neck controlling movement.

Working with a therapist or kinesiologist one-on-one, the injured patient rediscovers the comfort experienced with normal, healthy posture of the shoulder girdle and neck. As the upper thoracic and cervical spine approach neutral plane alignment, there is a lessening of the myofascial strain as the workload of the muscles reduces. The new neutral plane alignment and posture is also responsible for reducing the substantial fatigue associated with the chronic pain.

Daily attention to an exercise program and constant awareness of shoulder girdle posture are critical in the rehabilitation of whiplash-associated disorders. With the increasing level of comfort, patients are able to reintroduce aerobic programming which further contributes to the reduction of fatigue.

Aerobic programming and improvement in cardiovascular and respiratory function provide the elements of stamina, reducing the fatigue associated with chronic whiplash-associated disorders. Reduction of fatigue is a major contribution to reversing the collapse of the shoulder girdle and neck into the previously described sniff position.

It is also very important that exercise programming, like all the other therapies mentioned, be introduced in a very graduated fashion. Any attempts to accelerate the program will result in flare-ups and exacerbation, setting the entire rehabilitation process back.

It is also important to recognize that progress is not marked in a week, but more realistically in 1-2 months as might be expected in any fitness program. Celebrate the small successes and be consistent in your efforts. With these simple rules, you will likely find yourself on the straight road to recovery.

HOW MUCH TREATMENT IS ENOUGH?

"It's been such a long road to recovery; what if I stop treatment too soon?"

When should treatment stop? To answer this question, it may be helpful to divide patients with whiplash-associated injuries into three distinct groups:

1. mild or minor injuries achieving resolution within several weeks;
2. more significant injuries with or without predisposing degenerative problems such as osteoarthritis; and
3. injuries that show minimal improvement in level of comfort, even after various and ongoing therapeutic interventions.

GROUP 1

In the first group of whiplash patients, the answer is relatively clear-cut. It makes very little sense to continue with treatment in the absence of any complaint. Having resolved all symptoms, it is reasonable to expect that, if the whiplash patient remains symptom-free for a period of six months following completion of therapy, they can reasonably expect a favorable prognosis with little future sequelae.

That being said, if subjected to a significant hyperextension injury and given the body's natural healing process, one can expect resultant soft tissue scarring and a change from the original normal anatomy. The expectation of whether or not this individual may be more susceptible to further problems, in comparison to a person not involved in a whiplash accident, is certainly a consideration. **In other words, if they experience an additional whiplash injury, they are more likely to start in the second group.**

Some medical reviews have demonstrated that patients experiencing whiplash-associated injuries develop earlier osteoarthritic degenerative changes in their cervical spine when compared to a controlled peer group whom have not been subjected to whiplash injuries. These degenerative changes may cause a restricted range of motion of the cervical spine, which may be associated with discomfort. Degenerative changes of the intervertebral discs may also predispose them to premature rupture and herniation with additional associated problems.

> Unfortunately, there is no known medical or therapeutic intervention that will prevent the possibility of degenerative changes. The best strategy for fighting back is maintaining a full range of motion of the upper back and neck with diligent attention to core strength and posture. Following a prescribed exercise regime is vital.

GROUP 2

The second group of patients will have a more protracted course of treatment, possibly reflecting a more significant injury or underlying predisposing degenerative problem (such as prior trauma, arthritis, or osteoporosis) requiring additional time for healing. This group is characterized by a progressive but slower resolution pattern to their injury.

With the gradual resolution of symptoms with treatment, the time for conclusion of therapy becomes apparent to both the patient and the therapist. At this point, there will generally be a weaning-off process, whereby patients will be encouraged to extend time between visits and see how well they hold up on their own.

For maximum sustained recovery, it is expected that the whiplash patient will be instructed in a full exercise program, which they will diligently follow, both at home and possibly in a gym environment. In those individuals previously schooled, exercise may be conducted on their own. Otherwise, an attending kinesiologist or qualified exercise training professional is initially recommended.

Typically, because it is often a process of trial and error and individual tolerance, "biting off more than you can chew" in reintroducing normal activity and exercise may result in a two or three day flare-up of discomfort. If this occurs, the patient

"I'm scared to do anything anymore. What if I make it worse?"

should return for reassessment before their next scheduled appointment for treatment, at which time re-evaluation will indicate what further aspects in the treatment and management, if any, may require addressing.

Eventually, after trial and error, the patient becomes weaned from therapy and is encouraged to continue with the core exercise programming and the kinesthetic exercises to promote the shoulder girdle and cervical spine postural awareness that they have been taught during the rehabilitation process.

GROUP 3

The third group tends not to have such good fortune when it comes to resolution of symptoms. It may be that, in spite of best efforts and multiple therapies, this group reaches a level of stability in which further medical intervention does not improve level of comfort.

Those not reaching complete asymptomatic status with the standard therapies must make other decisions. Having read the previous chapters, most whiplash patients now have a concrete understanding of the underlying injury, the likely pain generators and the various therapies used in treatment and management.

> It is always reasonable to pursue the various available therapies in an attempt to resolve existing pain syndromes and improve level of function.

Remembering the *Rule of 6*, you can try any therapy for 6 visits. If failing to show any significant improvement in those visits, you are unlikely to show further improvement after 12 visits using the same modality of therapy.

Having achieved the best level of improvement, a visit to a pain clinic specializing in spinal disorders may be a reasonable option. Through the use of selective anesthetic blocks to specifically targeted apophyseal facet joints, nerve roots or intervertebral discs, it may be possible to isolate the pain generator and offer the patient an interventive treatment that will provide sustained relief from pain.

The process of determining the specific pain generator may take more than one scheduled visit, inasmuch as a systematic, step-by-step process is followed in a logical method, so as not to confuse which anatomical structure is the source of the pain syndrome. It is only by following such a disciplined process, that the patient can be offered a definitive management plan.

It is also regrettable, however, despite best treatment efforts, that a significant portion of patients may continue to report ongoing pain syndromes and limitation resulting in ongoing disability and impairment. This may be due to complicating accompanying factors including older age, pre-existing osteoarthritis and other infirmities or psychological impairments.

Medical treatment in these recalcitrant cases is likely to be considered palliative, designed to assist in management of the disability secondary to pain, in an effort to allow the patient to reach the best functioning level both relating to work environment and activities of daily living.

> Failure to show response to several therapies in the hands of experienced therapists, within a year of the injury, will likely result in a condition in which *time* more than any other factor, including different therapies, will be responsible for any change or improvement.

TAKING CHARGE

At this stage of the convalescence, the patient is very likely their own best physician. With the experience gained during a long rehabilitation, most patients have a fairly good idea which therapies best address their specific pain syndrome. There is no reason to limit these types of therapy, providing a good analysis of the risk/benefit ratio has been reasoned out.

HOW MUCH TREATMENT IS ENOUGH?

All patients should be encouraged to maintain as much of an active exercise program as they are capable. Medical research shows that retaining core strength and best postural alignment is the strongest indicator for achieving optimal outcome. When possible, walking and some types of swimming (in particular the backstroke) can be the simplest and least expensive forms of highly beneficial activity.

> Dependence on passive therapies may encourage a "victim mindset", which must always be guarded against.

Taking control of your life, even if compromised by impairment and disability, is critical to avoiding adoption of the "poor me syndrome". A positive mental attitude and involvement in life's activities will go a long way to preserving an optimistic outlook.

WHAT'S THE PROGNOSIS?

Although 80% of whiplash injuries will resolve their symptoms within 12 months following an accident, the other 20% will continue to have symptoms and 5% will be severely affected.

With over 10,000 English-language medical studies on whiplash, there has been a significant amount of research examining the long-term outcomes relating to whiplash-associated disorders. Although there may not be exact agreement on the figures, there is a general trend that is recognized as indicative of the consequences of this injury.

At the 6-month interval, a range between 19% to 60% of patients will continue to have significant complaints and 13% to 50% of this group will still not be able to perform their usual activities, may be absent from work or may otherwise restrict certain specific work duties.

As noted earlier, females and older individuals are 1.5 to 2 times more likely to suffer injury from whiplash than the general group and, therefore, are more predisposed to be still symptomatic at 6 months. This may possibly be attributed to lesser muscle mass or weakened muscle mass secondary to age or infirmity.

In addition to these factors, cervical spines that have pre-existing osteoarthritic changes or congenital anomalies (spines that show altered anatomical structure present from birth) also predispose patients to a less favorable prognosis.

Other associated conditions relating to the accident itself, or past medical histories that predispose to more severe injury and chronic symptoms, include:

- previous cervical spine injury
- presence of neck-pain symptoms prior to whiplash injury
- struck vehicle stationary at time of impact
- large striking vehicle (e.g., bus or truck)
- victim's head inclined or rotated at time of accident

There has been significant research to determine whether or not those patients likely to have a poorer prognosis can be recognized earlier. Certain characteristics noted within the first month post-injury may identify those most at risk.

Continuing to experience significant disability at 12 months, unfortunately, is not a good prognosticating factor. Following this group over the course of time demonstrates that 15 years post-injury, up to 70% may continue to experience symptoms.

Not surprisingly, there is a significant impact on the quality of life in these individuals with ongoing pain syndromes producing fatigue, sleep disturbances and other factors that may lead to ill health. Increasing sedentary behavior because of pain syndromes associated with physical activity, may lead to an increased risk for weight gain and all the attendant illnesses related to obesity, including diabetes and heart disease.

It is this group that are very likely drawn into the compensation process with insurance companies to ensure that they obtain the required resources to address necessary ongoing medical treatment, as well as adequate compensation for the loss in quality of life, financial earning capacity and future medical needs.

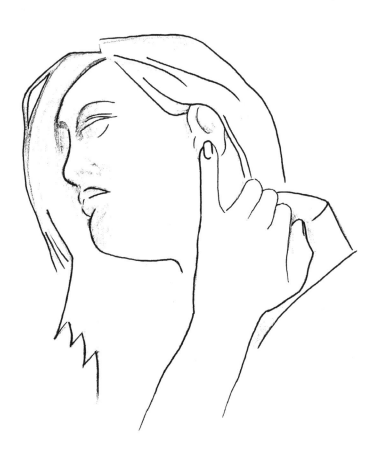

Characteristics That Tend Toward Poorer Prognosis

- need to attend emergency department post-accident due to significant injury

- initial high intensity of neck pain and headache

- pain that disturbs sleep

- higher levels of pain and disability within the first month

- evidence of psychological distress such as anxiety and fear

- evidence of nerve root irritation

- marked pain to light touch

- widespread hypersensitivity to blunt pressure

- hypersensitivity to heat and cold stimulation of affected tissues

- neuropsychological problems: dizziness, cognitive problems including attention and memory disturbances

Reading Notes:

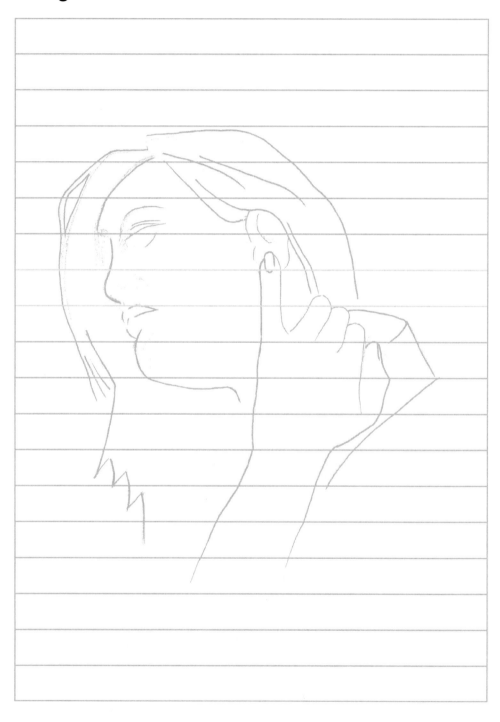

SECTION III
YOUR RIGHTS

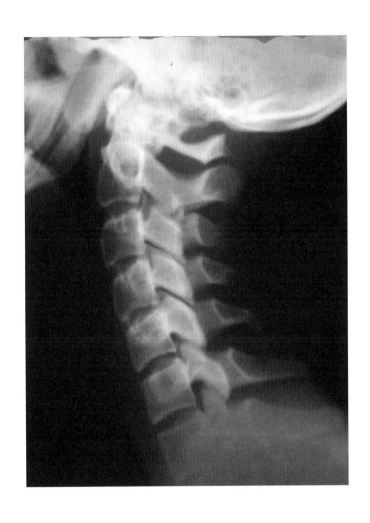

DOCUMENTING YOUR ACCIDENT AND YOUR INJURY

"It's all becoming a bit of a blur…"

The sooner you can sit down and document the details of your motor vehicle accident and the course of events that followed, the better. All memories tend to blur with time. This documentation is especially important if you anticipate difficulties settling your claim with your insurance company, or if you end up in court to negotiate a settlement.

In addition to outlining the facts for your legal counsel, the details of the accident will be critically important to both your treating therapists as well as any professional medical experts that you may attend in preparation for the negotiation process of your award settlement. Many of these details will be indicative of the forces involved in the collision, as well as the biomechanics of the injury process itself.

Checklists have been included within this book (see Appendix B) for your reference. You can also visit *www.ChronicBackPainClinic.com* to download hardcopies for completion.

DOCUMENTING YOUR ACCIDENT AND YOUR INJURY

Preparing a document with the following details, will be extremely helpful and an enormous timesaver during the course of future interviews (many professional fees are by-the-hour, so time is definitely money). It may also be useful to send it prior to initial appointments, giving that professional an opportunity to review the details and prepare any additional questions.

Ultimately, this completed document shows you are organized, you understand the biomechanics relating to the whiplash-associated injury, and you are seriously in pursuit of a solution to your problem.

DOCUMENTING YOUR ACCIDENT

GENERAL INFORMATION

- Your name
- Date and time of injury
- Address of collision
- Estimated damage to the vehicle
- Police or emergency vehicles attending collision site
- Brief description of how the crash happened

INVOLVED VEHICLES

- Model, year and make of your vehicle
- Model, year and make of other involved vehicle(s)

Size and weight are important. Comments as to whether or not the involved vehicles were subcompact, compact, mid-size, full-size, pickup, larger than 1 ton, towing or carrying cargo should be documented.

ESTIMATED CRASH SPEEDS

The estimated speed of your vehicle and others' gives some indication of the forces involved in the collision. It is also important to know whether or not the vehicles involved were stopped, slowing down, gaining speed or moving at a steady speed.

WHAT WERE YOU DOING AT THE TIME OF THE CRASH?

Your awareness of the moment of collision is also pertinent in terms of the injuries experienced.

- Were you aware of the impending crash and, if so, were you braced or relaxed?
- Were you wearing a seat belt?
- Were you holding onto the steering wheel at the time of impact?

The position of your head is also important: was it inclined or rotated? For example, were you looking in the rearview or side mirror at the time of the collision or were you looking straightforward? Had you turned your head to speak to someone in the back seat or were you looking down to adjust the radio?

WHAT DID YOUR CAR DO AFTER IMPACT?

What happened after the collision is also important.

- Did your car move forward? If so, did it move forward in a straight line or did it spin?

- Did it hit anything?
- Was it hit multiple times? If so, what were the circumstances of each impact?
- Did it flip or roll?
- How did your vehicle ultimately come to rest?

WHAT HAPPENED TO YOU IN THE COLLISION?

With the duration of the accident lasting only milliseconds, it can be difficult to be aware of all the circumstances of your body before, during and after the collision. It is important, however, to recall as many details as possible. Whether or not they seem relevant to you at the present time, they may have significance at a later time upon questioning.

- Did your head or shoulder make contact with the side window or door frame?
- If there was another occupant in the vehicle, did you make contact with them?
- Were you struck by any cargo in the vehicle?
- Did your knee(s) make contact with the dash, steering column, or seat in front of you?
- Were you aware of bracing or jamming your foot/feet prior to the accident?
- Were you aware of bracing yourself with your hands prior to the accident?

WERE YOU AWARE OF ANY BRUISING OR SORENESS FROM YOUR SEATBELT?

- Were any parts within the vehicle broken, bent or damaged?
- Was there any damage to the steering wheel, side window, seat frame, knee bolster or rearview mirror?
- Was there any damage to the side doors? Were you able to exit from them?

ABOUT YOUR HEAD RESTRAINTS

- If your vehicle was equipped with head rests, were they fixed or movable?
- Estimate the distance between the back of your head and the front of the head restraint.
- Indicate the position of the headrest:
  - level with your shoulder blades, neck
  - lower height at the back of your head
  - midway height at the back of your head
  - midway height at the top of the back of your head

AFTER THE ACCIDENT

- Did an emergency vehicle attend the scene?
- Did you receive any immediate attention at the accident scene?
- Did you go to an emergency department after the accident? (name of hospital, date, time, and attending physicians)

DID YOU LEAVE THE ACCIDENT SCENE BY YOURSELF OR WERE YOU ACCOMPANIED BY ANOTHER PERSON?

- Were you hospitalized or observed in the emergency ward for a period of time?
- Did you have any tests or x-rays?
- Did you have any cuts, abrasions, lacerations or stitches?
- Were you given any prescriptions by the emergency room doctor when you left? (names of drugs and dosage)

WHEN DID YOU FIRST SEE A DOCTOR?

- When did you first notice symptoms following your injury? Immediately after the accident, within hours, within days? Be specific!
- If you delayed getting medical attention following the accident for your symptoms, why?
  - unable to schedule doctors appointment
  - no transportation
  - work/home schedule conflicts
  - self-treated

SUSTAINED HEAD INJURY

- Did you lose consciousness or black out for any length of time?
- Have you lost any of your memory for the timeframe prior to the head injury?

- Has your memory been different in any way since the injury?
- Did you have any lumps or bruises after the head injury? If so, where and how severely?
- Have you had any head injuries in your past, including child-hood?
- Did you have any x-rays, CAT scans or MRIs taken of your head since the accident?

Symptoms That May Relate Specifically to Whiplash-Associated Injuries

- Headache
- Dizziness
- Tinnitus (ear ringing)
- Blurry vision
- Balance problems
- Loss of coordination
- Pain/difficulty swallow-ing
- Wrist/hand/finger pain and/or numbness
- Jaw pain
- Neck pain/soreness
- Neck stiffness
- Shoulder pain/stiffness
- Arm pain/tingling/ numbness

- Weakness in arms/legs
- Upper/mid back pain
- Chest wall pain (rib or ribs)
- Low back pain/ soreness
- Hip pain
- Leg pain
- Leg numbness/tingling
- Shooting pain down legs
- Knee pain
- Ankle/foot pain
- Other changes in comfort or proper function

ABILITY TO WORK

- Were you unable to work following the injury? If so, list dates and hours missed.
- Have you had to change your work duties since your injury because of limitations? Describe the changes necessary.

ABILITY TO MAINTAIN NORMAL ACTIVITIES

- Have your normal activities changed? If so, what and how?
- Are you able to care for your children in typical fashion?

DOCUMENTING YOUR TREATMENT

Often by the time patients with whiplash-associated injury realize that adjudication will be required for claims settlement, a considerable amount of time may have passed. It is very common for whiplash patients to have received treatment from several therapists and been evaluated by more than one medical doctor.

Documenting the treatment(s) received in the order in which they are administered will contribute important information to the comprehensive medical record. Also document if you are/were receiving more than one therapy concurrently.

DOCUMENTING YOUR ACCIDENT AND YOUR INJURY

The following information should be included for each therapist or doctor seen, in chronological order.

- Name of doctor/therapist/center
- Addresses, contact info (phone, fax, email)
- Dates of treatment
- Type of therapy (physiotherapy, massage, chiropractic, etc.)
- Number of visits
- X-rays: what body parts; name of x-ray clinic
- MRI / CAT scan
- Other diagnostic tests completed or ordered
- Medications prescribed
- Types of therapy: massage, heat or ice packs, ultrasound, diathermy, interferential current, acupuncture, exercise programming, etc.
- Results of therapy:
    - helped during treatment but symptoms returned when treatment stopped
    - treatment helped and improvement remained when treatment stopped
    - no benefit
    - made symptoms worse

Reading Notes:

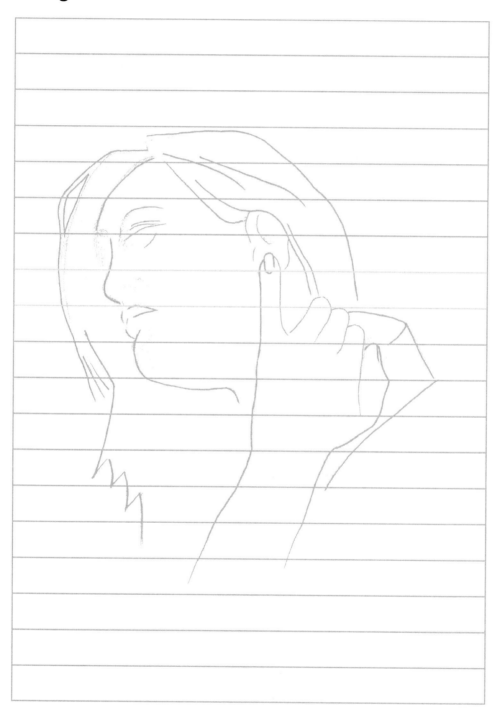

UNDERSTANDING YOUR OPPONENT:
PUT ON YOUR INSURANCE ADJUSTER HAT

"The insurance company is making me feel worse!"

Other than in circumstances in which a whiplash injury requires little need for medical intervention, it is quite likely that you will need to deal with at least one insurance company. In some cases, this will be the same insurance company that will be fixing your car. In other jurisdictions, especially with those individuals who have additional third-party coverage, additional insurance companies may also be involved.

Your contact at the insurance company will likely be an insurance adjuster, but in cases of serious injury, you may have a case manager assigned to your case to assist you in coordinating your rehabilitative care. This is unlikely to have occurred with a straightforward case of whiplash-associated injury, unless there are associated cognitive disabilities subsequent to your injuries.

In any dealings with insurance adjusters, it is always wisest to plan what you are going to say in a concise manner, getting to the point quickly, without elaborate discourse. You should be keeping notes of any conversations and contact that you have

Remember: *your insurance company is not your friend.* As much as the insurance adjuster may appear empathetic, it is in the best economic interests of the insurance company to limit the claim of damages.

with your adjuster, *because you can be absolutely certain they will be.* Your record-keeping skills may place you in good stead in the future, should any of these details come into question.

If your insurance company has adopted a policy that low-velocity-impact accidents are unlikely to be associated with any significant compensable injuries, you may find the insurance representative assigned to your case is less than helpful—*or denies your claim outright.*

It is useful to visit your attending physician prior to any contact with your insurance company, so you can inform the agent that you have been examined by your doctor and your injuries have been objectively documented. The insurance representative can then be advised that they are at liberty to write your physician for further information should they wish—a likelihood that will occur in any case.

This brings up a very important point. Having filed an insurance claim for your whiplash injury, you generally give up your right to doctor-patient confidentiality; at least in respect to all of your office visits that relate to your present injury, or any prior visits in your medical history that may be broadly relevant to problems related to upper back or neck health issues, or to other causes of disability. This means that the insurance company has the right to subpoena and examine treatment and clinical records and, in fact, contact your doctor to ask questions about any matter relevant to your claim.

If there are parts of your medical record that you do not wish to be released to the insurance company, especially if you believe they do not specifically relate to your present muscle skeletal problems, you may wish to retain legal counsel right from the onset.

Some insurance companies will go on fishing expeditions, delving into your past medical history, in an attempt to find information that may be helpful in limiting or denying your claim. By obtaining legal counsel, you may make application to the court to limit the medical information released to the insurance company to relevant materials as defined by the court.

PAYING FOR TREATMENT: WHO OPENS THEIR WALLET FIRST?

In the end, if your insurance claim is accepted, you can expect to be reimbursed for all reasonable costs of therapy in the management of your rehabilitation.

Whether or not you have to first personally pay individual therapists may depend on both the therapist's and the insurance company's policies. Some insurance companies will only directly pay for certain types of therapy (e.g., massage or physiotherapy). If you have decided that acupuncture is your choice of therapy, you may have to pay for it yourself with the expectation of reimbursement at the time of settlement of your claim. You may also find that insurance companies will only pay for a fixed number of visits for a particular therapy, regardless of the recommendations of your therapist or physician.

Almost all insurance companies have a special criterion for low income-eligible claimants or other specially designated groups. With specific documentation and written physician referral, you may find that the insurance company will accept direct billing from the therapist you are attending, if the therapy has been recommended by your doctor. This may also apply to fitness and exercise programming and even gym memberships if recommended by your physician or therapist for specific rehabilitative purposes.

Some therapy clinics have policies not to deal with outside parties and will expect payment directly from their clients at the time service has been rendered. Under these circumstances, again you must pay for your own care and arrange for reimbursement of costs at the time of settlement of claim with your insurance company.

Some motor vehicle accident insurance companies have a special reserve benefit portion, specifically earmarked for payment of medical rehabilitation and related expenses. These funds, which exist separately from the claim process for damages, may be used for payment of specific therapeutic benefits that may relate to therapies, prescription drugs, medical supplies and equipment, hospital beds and in-home attendant care.

Accessing these funds may require the services of legal counsel, as they are normally reserved for extended rehabilitation costs that often fall out of the normal expected payment capabilities of the average claimant. If you find your treatment costs stretching your budget, asking about access to this funding may be a reasonable option.

When Insurance May Be Void

There are certain circumstances in which any claim against your insurance company may be void, regardless of the severity of injuries that you have experienced. These policies are normally outlined in your insurance agreement.

Situations that may exclude you from insurance coverage may involve hit-and-run accidents, being under the influence of alcohol or drugs at the time of the accident, or if your insurance had expired when the accident occurred. In other cases, insurance exclusion may apply if you are liable and causative of the accident.

If the conditions surrounding your motor vehicle accident are complicated by issues such as these, it is very likely that you would benefit from the assistance of qualified legal counsel.

WHAT YOU SAY
CAN AND WILL BE USED AGAINST YOU

"Should I get a lawyer?"

Many whiplash victims find themselves jolted as they observe adversarial practices of insurance companies.

First and foremost, do not be surprised to find the insurance company denying or minimizing your claim. Their starting point will likely be, "There is little or no injury and, therefore, no disability and impairment."

So, should you get a lawyer? The short answer to this question is: it depends. If your injuries were limited, with little need for medical management, and your attending physician has given you assurances that you can expect recovery to pre-

Note: No one should settle while still experiencing adverse symptoms due to the accident.

NEVER settle prior to six months post-injury.

83

accident status within a reasonable timeframe of, perhaps, six months, it may not be worth the effort.

Unless you are prepared to pay the hourly billing fee of your legal counsel, you will likely be entering into a contingency fee agreement with your lawyer. This means that, instead of hourly billing for your lawyer's services, he or she will expect to be paid between 15% and 33.3% of your settlement or court award.

If you are satisfied with the offer the insurance company has placed before you, it makes little sense to consider legal representation that will ultimately reduce the total amount you receive.

If you have missed an inordinate amount of work or incurred significant costs relating to medical treatment of your injuries, or if your symptoms have not resolved within 12 to 18 months of your injury, you may wish to retain legal counsel to obtain the best representation in settling your claim.

Most lawyers who specialize in injury law are willing to see you for a free initial appointment. There is no harm in seeing one or more lawyers before deciding whether it would be in your best interest to hire a lawyer early on or to wait until the insurance company makes you an offer. The lawyer does not necessarily have to tell the insurance company right away that you have, in fact, hired them.

Statistics provide a strong argument for obtaining professional legal counsel. When you look at the statistics of whiplash injuries, one-third of whiplash victims will retain legal counsel to represent them in their dealings with the insurance company. When you look at the total amounts of claim dollars paid out by insurance companies to whiplash victims, two-thirds are paid to people who have obtained legal counsel, keeping in mind that the more severe the injury, the more likely the victim is to hire a lawyer.

CHOOSING THE RIGHT LAWYER FOR YOU

Finding a good lawyer is much like finding any good professional, whether it is a doctor, dentist or psychologist. The issue relates not only to their knowledge but also to your ability to relate to them. If you find your lawyer empathetic, understanding, forthcoming and available when you require them—*and with plenty of experience going to trial*—you have probably made an excellent choice.

Most professionals take pride in their work and make efforts to keep up with the knowledge base referable to their clients' needs. If there are aspects of your case which they feel may need special attention, it is not unreasonable for your lawyer to ask for outside help to assist in the presentation of your case. The key to any professional relationship is your trust in their judgment and your comfort level in their presence.

Most certainly, you should expect them to have a successful history of representing other clients with similar needs. Most reputable legal representatives are more than happy to supply you with examples of their work. Some may even have testimonial letters on file or be willing to allow you to talk to previous clients if they have obtained the client's permission to do so.

> You have the right to ask your lawyer to resolve your claim sooner rather than later, if time, not a maximum possible settlement, is more important to you. *You're in charge.*

It is very important that you feel comfortable with the legal representative you retain—*your relationship with this person will likely continue for some time.* If your injuries are significant and your recovery is slow, it is probable that the negotiation process before settlement will take place up to 18 months to 3 years from the date of the accident.

It is also important that your legal counsel have a good understanding of the biomechanics of whiplash-associated injury, the natural history of recovery, the available treatments options and the prognosis associated with your outcome. While they should not replace the role of your physician or rehabilitation therapists, if you find you know more about whiplash than they do, you should seek better legal representation.

DISCUSSING COSTS WITH YOUR LAWYER

Clearly defined agreements make for good professional relationships. It makes very good sense to clarify what the costs of retaining a professional will be and to fully understand how the professional relationship will move forward before you get into it. Forewarned is forearmed!

The last thing you need is a "falling out" with your lawyer, in the middle of what tends to be a stressful process.

Discuss in detail with your lawyer—*before you hire them*—the likelihood that you will be reimbursed for legal fees and expenses such as expert witnesses.

The Cost of Expert Witnesses

In preparation of your case, there will be the need to hire professional expert witnesses to provide evidence of your claim for damages. Although these professionals are specifically discussed in a later chapter, it is important to realize that the costs of these consultations and the resulting expert reports may vary from several hundred dollars to over $10,000 each, depending on the depth of study and detail the medical expert will require.

WHAT YOU SAY CAN AND WILL BE USED AGAINST YOU

Payment to these professionals will be expected when their service is rendered. It is important for you to come to an agreement with your legal counsel as to who will pay for these reports. It is customary that your legal representative pay for these services as you go along; however, the ultimate settling of disbursements differs between jurisdictions and lawyers.

Note: There will likely be interest charges applied by your lawyer for funds advanced in payment of these reports and charges. You can negotiate this, so be sure the rate of interest is reasonable.

In some cases in some jurisdictions, if you win your case and the court considers the money spent on the medical examinations and reports critical to your defense, the disbursement of payment for these examinations and reports will be covered under costs and not deducted from your award settlement.

On the other hand, if a specific examination and expert report were considered unnecessary in establishing your defense, these costs may be excluded.

It is also possible that, on the recommendation of your legal representative, you may attend a medical expert who produces an unfavorable report to your case. Under those circumstances, even though the costs for the report have been incurred, your lawyer will choose not to include the information in your legal presentation.

Under these circumstances, particularly when your lawyer suggested the specific test, consultation or medical legal report, you may wish to have determined beforehand what percentage of these fees for unused evidence your legal representative will be responsible for, since it will otherwise come directly out of your settlement.

In special cases in some jurisdictions, if the court decides to award you with a compensation package greater than the insurance company had initially offered you, the court may award "double costs" to you. What this means is the court will order the insurance company to pay you double the disbursement costs required for you to prepare your case. Representing a penalty to the insurance company for their low offer in compensation for your injuries, it represents a windfall for you.

If you have anticipated this possibility, you should take it into consideration in your early discussions with your legal counsel, determining whether or not this part of the award will fall within the contingency fee agreement.

> Be aware of the laws and regulations as they apply in your particular jurisdiction. What may be standard practice in one jurisdiction, may not be so in another. Don't assume anything. Be specific with your lawyer.

In situations where either the insurance company or you initiate an appeal of the trial court's decision, the arrangements for ongoing legal fees and expenses should be agreed to beforehand. It is not unusual for contingency fee agreements to change under appeal circumstances. Often, an hourly rate may apply. The risk of winning or losing an appeal is considerably different from the original action, given the risk that both parties may put in considerable time without compensation.

If your whiplash-associated disorder has not resolved and your medical caregivers estimate you have reached maximum medical improvement (MMI), it will be necessary for you to convince either the insurance company or the court to the extent of your impairment and disability.

WHAT YOU SAY CAN AND WILL BE USED AGAINST YOU

In clinical practice, those victims of whiplash injury who still have significant physical pain at 18-months post-injury, in spite of best efforts at clinical intervention, have very likely reached MMI.

MMI is a term used to indicate that any further recovery is only likely to occur over an extended period of time—*if at all*. Despite medical intervention, the condition in question can no longer be anticipated to improve within a reasonable degree of medical certainty, implying that the injury is permanent and unchanging. How this legally translates into impairment and disability needs to be subjected to objective testing to fairly appraise the individual's compromised existence.

Determining the level of disability and impairment is generally defined by obtaining past medical records outlining the original diagnosis and treatment to date, arranging specific medical testing to quantify the injuries, as well as arranging appointments with various medical experts to complete examinations and prepare specific reports. In these reports, the medical experts outline their clinical findings and state their own conclusions as to the level of disability and impairment imposed by the injuries.

Reading Notes:

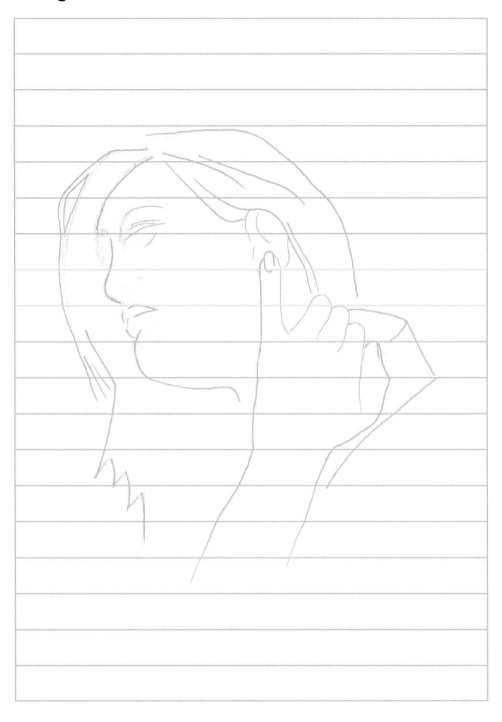

YOURS, MINE, AND OURS:
MEDICAL EXPERTS AND THE LAW

"Who can I trust?"

A medical expert is recognized as one who has, by experience, acquired special knowledge of the subject about which he or she will testify. A prognosis is a medical opinion as to the likely course and outcome of an injury or disease. Determining a whiplash-injury prognosis is best described as an "art" or "skill" rather than a science, thus creating the possibility of conflicting opinions among medical experts.

The medical expert's responsibility is to provide an opinion of a possible outcome that falls within the "criteria of certainty" *—very specifically applied in legal circumstances to mean greater than a 50% probability.*

The medical expert must take many variables into consideration including changes over time, modification by age, alteration of present medical status by possible further intervention, additional medical complications as well as emotional stress and neuropsychiatric impact.

91

The best medical experts tend to rely on information that is well accepted by their peers. They avoid novel interpretation of data and assist the court in appreciating the technical variables under question. It is important for the expert to be consistent in the methodology upon which their opinions are formed, and to present the information in an impartial manner, without advocacy or the drawing of conclusions that fall within the jurisdiction of the court.

> The last thing you wish to do is get upset and give the insurance company's examining doctor reason to believe your behavior is emotional or indicative of overreacting. Your day will come in court, so keep your composure and maintain the expected civility.

To be less than this reduces the effectiveness of the testimony and often creates disfavor to the presenting side. This is especially so if the presentation is obscure, pretentious or technically confusing.

Unfortunately, this defines medical experts in a perfect world. Be forewarned: not only does your legal representative get to choose medical experts for your side, the insurance company gets to do the same.

These experts have been hand-picked by the insurance company and, unfortunately, for a very specific reason: they tend to find in favor of the insurance company. The only thing that you as the injured party can do is not take it personally and recognize that this is just part of the adversarial legal process.

The best advice when you see these arranged medical consultants is to stick to your story, be cooperative during the history-taking process and do not try to magnify your complaint. Whatever you say or do, you are unlikely to favorably influence these examiners in any case.

All groups of evaluating experts will likely include tools or instruments in the process of their examination, that would detect the examinee's efforts to influence the observer's interpretation, suggesting exaggeration of their disability.

Known generically as "organic signs", these behaviors are, at best, interpreted as secondary-gain unconscious efforts representing sick roles and illness behaviors. These illness behaviors produce beneficial gains in the day-to-day life activities of the individual involved (e.g., delaying return to work, enjoying the extra attention gained by illness). At worst, they represent fictitious malingering for the purpose of defrauding a system designed to protect them.

Medical experts relying on investigative instruments in measuring functional, cognitive or neuropsychiatric impairment are expected to be well-versed in the weaknesses and strengths of the tools they employ in their assessments and should be familiar with the current clinical literature in their area of expertise, in order to withstand challenges during examination.

SUPPORTING YOUR CASE WITH OBJECTIVE DATA

In support of the whiplash victim, there are a number of clinical studies and evaluations that can be undertaken to quantify the degree of disability and impairment of each individual client.

Working together with your attending doctors and therapists, your legal counsel will methodically gather the needed evidence to support your disability and claim. There are a number of medical assessments that may be required to obtain the necessary objective information to substantiate your level of disability.

Medical Legal Report: It is common to obtain medical legal reports from the attending physicians, chiropractors and therapists to outline the clinical status of the patient prior to the injury, the effect of the injury in the immediate post-accident phase, the present disability and impairment, and the expectation of future impairment as a result of the injuries. If this report suggests that future impairment or disability is expected, there are a number of avenues available to qualify and quantify the degree of disability and impairment for which compensation should be sought.

Neurological Evaluation: Clear-cut cases of obvious neurological damage are the easiest, inasmuch as the issue is not the existence of, but rather the extent and implications of the neurological damage. Damage to nervous tissue can be demonstrated through radiological examination where disruption of normal anatomy can be clearly shown. Disruption of intervertebral discs, fractures or dislocations with nerve root impingement, and compromise of nerve function corroborated through objective nerve conduction and electromyographic studies, all point to neurological damage. Referrals for these studies are readily available to all attending physicians. The implication of impairment and disability in terms of its impact on activities of daily living and vocation may require additional assessment.

Rehabilitative Medical Assessment and Evaluation: Undertaken by specialized medical doctors called physiatrists, the objective of this assessment is to determine (using accepted standardized methodologies) permanent impairment and the impact it has on daily living and work. Having identified the pertinent medical diagnoses, impairments, functional limitations and the impact of the medical impairment, this _employability assessment_ involves evaluation of the individual's ability to perform their specific job without endangering themselves or others in the work environment, or the workplace itself.

Functional Capacity Evaluation (FCE): Conducted by specialized physical/occupational therapists, FCEs comprise batteries of tests designed to make repeated musculoskeletal observations as to range of motion, muscle strength testing, and material-handling abilities including lifting capacities, pushing or pulling capacities and carrying capacities. They also test postural tolerances for walking, standing, sitting, squatting, kneeling, reaching, bending, and the ability to negotiate stairs and ramps. With a thorough working knowledge of the expectations of the workplace and home environment, the examining therapist provides a practical assessment of the ability of the individual to function in specific environments.

Chronic Pain Impairment Evaluation: Pain management physicians can objectively determine the presence or absence of pain using controlled, double-blinded, cervical apophyseal facet joint blocks with local anesthetics, which may be helpful in presenting supportive evidence. However, only you know how much it really hurts. Pain and suffering exist as a manifestation of extended consciousness and thus can only be inferred by the observer *without supportive direct objective measurement*. Therefore, at least some degree of subjective patient self-reporting is required to determine the real impact on coping abilities, activities of daily living, environmental stresses, and capacity for work. Through the use of batteries of psychometric tests, psychologists trained in pain assessment can evaluate the psychosocial and behavioral variables that measure the levels of interference with everyday life due to the pain and effective distress. The testing parameters recognize that individuals vary in their capability to adapt and cope, and measure with reliable internal consistency coefficients, the impact of pain and suffering on the performance of daily activity.

Neuropsychiatric Evaluation: Mild Traumatic Brain Injury (MTBI) may represent either a focal or diffuse pattern of neurocognitive deficits. Testing must comprehensively examine sensory and perceptual processes, motor functions, central processing functions, executive abilities, and intellectual and academic abilities. Through the use of multiple tests, this battery of assessments provides a reliable vector of evidence with inter-rater reliability (the extent to which two or more observers agree). These assessments are time consuming and costly, but in appropriate subjects are critical to determine the future needs of the compromised individual by identifying neurocognitive deficits and providing realistic expectations of recovery.

Psychiatric Evaluation: Post Traumatic Stress Disorder (PTSD) is commonly recognized following motor vehicle accidents. PTSD requires intensive psychiatric and psychometric evaluation to differentiate it from other psychiatric diagnoses and comorbid illnesses (concurrent chronic illnesses). Presence of symptoms at 21-days post-accident has been found to be a significant predictor of persistent symptoms at 12-month follow-up. Whereas most of us would likely admonish ourselves to "pull up our socks and get on with it", these individuals may become significantly psychologically destabilized due to an underlying vulnerability providing grounds for ongoing impairment and disability.

Crash Biomechanics Evaluation: In situations where the magnitude of symptom presentation may not be in keeping with the observable damage to the vehicle, it may be necessary to employ accident reconstruction engineers to assess the impact severity in relationship to the threshold for injury. This group of professionals has graduate-level training in both medical and engineering studies providing scientific expertise in assessing the impact of mechanical forces and the resultant disruption of biological tissues.

Future Medical Costs and Income Losses Assessment: When impairment and disability are identified, a compensatory monetary value must be assigned to address the long-term economic and societal implications of an injury. Having determined that the whiplash patient has reached maximum medical improvement (MMI) and there is likelihood of a permanent impairment rating, it becomes critical to assign an economic loss and cost when causality can be directly linked, within a medical certainty, to the motor vehicle accident in question. *Legal counsel should be cautious in asking medical experts to predict future medical costs and economic losses unless they are qualified to do so.* Should such information be necessary, close operation with actuarial experts should be employed in creating well-outlined and accurate estimations to stand up to examination scrutiny.

If your legal counsel presents your case with reliance on objective findings, it is likely to result in your favor. If your case is presented with minimal supporting substantive medical evidence, the insurance company's core strategy need be little more than innuendo and implication that you are exaggerating your symptoms and that the court should minimize any compensation awarded to you.

Placing the onus solely on the credibility of your story fails to bring to the court all the assessment tools available to objectively prove your case. By applying the assessment instruments of the scientific community to the question of impairment and disability, you increase the likelihood of the court coming to a fair and equitable judgment, awarding you the appropriate compensation to which you are due.

Reading Notes:

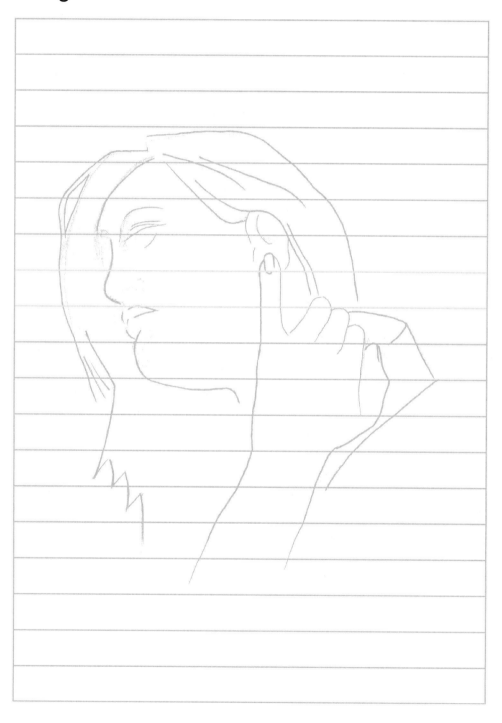

SECTION IV
REBUILDING YOUR LIFE

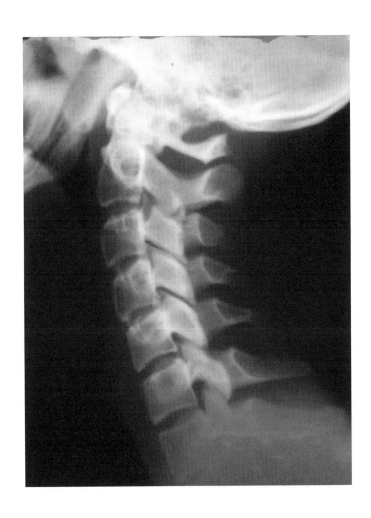

REBUILDING YOUR LIFE: *THIS TOO SHALL PASS*

"Whiplash consumed my life. How do I move on?"

It has been estimated that symptoms may improve 20% to 30% with the completion of the negotiation and judicial process.

Many people find the process of pursuing a financial settlement following a whiplash injury a constant reminder of the accident itself. Any psychological stress you may have associated with your accident tends to be kept at the surface, with very little opportunity for emotional wounds to heal. Constant reminders of disabling symptoms, pain, disruptions to daily living and financial hardship subsequent to the accident cannot be conducive to optimum healing.

Now that the settlement process is complete, you have your chance at closure and can begin looking to the future knowing you have concluded at least one unpleasant chapter of your life. While some may have ongoing therapy in their pursuit of maximum recovery, many others, given the extended length of time required to conclude their settlement process, have already been advised by their attending physicians that maximum medical improvement (MMI) has been reached. Further improvement from this time forward will likely be attributed to time rather than any specific therapeutic intervention.

Under these circumstances, most patients can competently become their own doctors. No one knows your body and its responses better than you. *You can trust yourself.* If you find that a specific therapy applied at intervals produces a level of comfort that permits you to function at a higher level in terms of your work and leisure, by all means apply that therapy at your discretion.

The most important thing to remember, however, is that some therapies may have risks attached to them; it is necessary to have a good understanding of the risks and benefits associated with your therapy of choice. Just as reading this book has educated you regarding your whiplash, it is wise to continue to educate yourself on all aspects of your treatment and recovery.

Alternatively, some may stop therapeutic intervention entirely, choosing to live within their newly established limits of activity. In most cases—*regardless of activity*—level of comfort is generally the only thing in jeopardy. Apart from a two to three day flare-up of symptoms, you will not likely do any real harm to your ongoing recovery. With this realization, most people will quickly come to their own conclusions as to the level of activity and risk with which they are willing to live.

THE RISK OF INACTIVITY

Keeping up your level of fitness, especially central core fitness supporting the shoulder girdle and upper spinal posture, is critical to maintaining a level of comfort and sustaining the gains made with therapy. *Use it or lose it!*

The greatest risk to optimum recovery is ongoing inactivity and a *victim mentality*. While it is true that you may not be able to resume all the activities with the same vigor and stamina that you did prior to the accident, a positive mental attitude will go a long way in supporting recovery to your best level of functioning.

THE TRIUMPHANT TRIO: CORE STRENGTH, AEROBIC FITNESS, AND PERFECT POSTURE

If you've read this book, you are clearly a proactive individual not willing to sit back and wait for someone else to lead your recovery. That same attitude will serve you well in rebuilding your life to pre-accident status—*or better!*

Prior to your injury, you may have taken your health and fitness for granted. Now that you have experienced recovery from a whiplash-associated disorder, you may be far more motivated to strive for maximum health and vitality. To achieve it following whiplash, you must give priority to three specific categories of fitness: core strength, aerobic fitness, and perfect posture.

Core strength is far more than strong abdominals. The "core" consists of supporting muscles that run the entire length of the torso, keeping the spine, pelvis, and shoulder girdle aligned, comfortable, and able to function appropriately. A strong core can be your back's best defense.

Pursuing *aerobic fitness* does not mean you have to start running marathons! Going for an early morning stroll or a brisk walk after dinner are both appropriate techniques for increasing aerobic health. Technically speaking, aerobic fitness increases oxygen in the bloodstream and delivers maximum levels to the muscles. Activities that increase heart rate and respiration are key.

Benefits to aerobic fitness extend far beyond the physical. While increased energy, stamina, and strength are all part of the package, so is a better mental outlook. Aerobic fitness has shown to be a very useful tool in the fight against depression.

As with any new aerobic training program, particularly in recovery from whiplash, it is advised that you see your physician first. They can discuss heart rate increases, duration and frequency of the aerobic activities that are appropriate for you. A simple rule of thumb is 30-minutes, a minimum of three times per week, at a respiratory level that challenges you but still allows you to continue a conversation (if you're panting too hard to speak, you may need to slow down!).

Sit up straight! It turns out our mothers were right. **Perfect posture** is conducive to eliminating back pain altogether, whether it be whiplash-induced or the result of almost any back injury. And it's far easier than you may think. In the book *Healing Chronic Back Pain: Seven Steps to Perfect Posture,* you will find a straight-forward, no-nonsense approach to achieving and maintaining healthy, pain-free posture.

Safe and Healthy Choices for Fitness After Whiplash Recovery

- Ballroom dancing
- Swimming
- Brisk walking
- Jogging
- Cycling (recumbent best)
- Yoga
- Golf (walking with push cart)
- Curling, bowling

For more information visit
www.HealingChronicBackPain.com.

Simply becoming aware of your posture and self-correcting through-out the normal activities of your day can deliver enormous gains in relieving any number of back complaints.

You are undoubtedly anxious to get on with your life. Consider the follow-ing activities and see how quickly your recovery from whiplash can go from a debilitating mix of pain and frustration to an invigorating mix of fun and fitness.

EXERCISE THERAPIES IN
WHIPLASH REHABILITATION

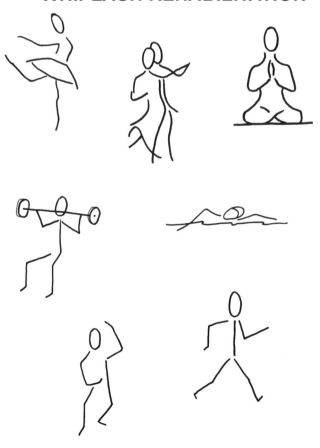

Reading Notes:

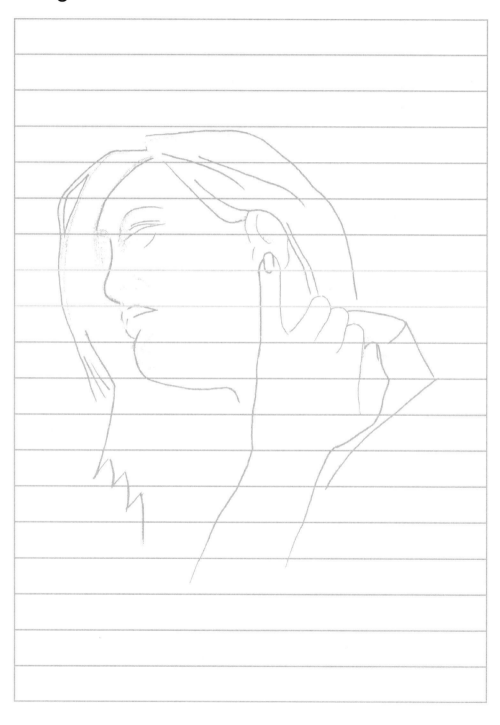

SECTION V

ONE-STOP WHIPLASH REFERENCE GUIDE

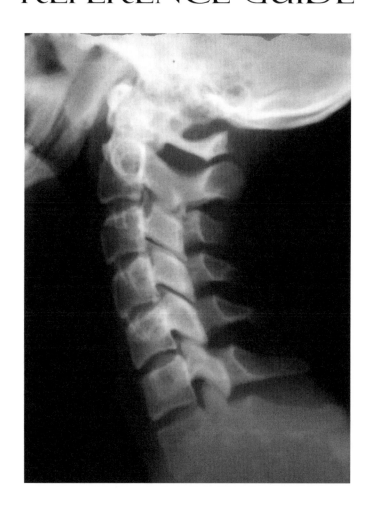

APPENDIX A: GLOSSARY

Acquired scoliosis

An acquired side-bending or lateral rotation of the spine that was not present at birth and is often representative of spasm of paraspinal muscles, more marked on one side of the spine than the other. Often seen in x-rays, it represents increased muscle tone often as a response to injury.

Activator techniques

A chiropractic technique using a hand-held adjusting instrument, which gives consistent low-force high-speed chiropractic adjustments.

Analgesics (pain killers)

Medications prescribed by physicians or obtained from over-the-counter sources including pharmacies and health food stores, for the purpose of relieving pain.

Anesthetic blocks

See spinal nerve root blocks, epidural injections.

Anterior muscles

When referring to anatomical areas, anterior refers to the front side of the body, as opposed to posterior which refers to the back side of the body.

Antidepressants (tricyclics) A class of drugs used for their ability to effect muscle contraction in whiplash-associated disorders, producing relaxation of spastic muscle groups. They also have the effect of improving sleep patterns and reducing fatigue.

Anti-inflammatories

A class of drugs identified by their anti-inflammatory properties. Also called NSAIDs (nonsteroidal anti-inflammatory drugs) they may be available from over-the-counter sources as well as physician pre-scriptions. A number of natural herbs are also identified to have anti-inflammatory qualities, includ-ing ginger, hyssop, tumeric and ar-nica montana. One of the oldest drugs identified to have anti-inflammatory abilities is Aspirin isolated from willow bark.

Apophyseal joint (vertebral)

Referred to by many different terms including facet joint, apophy-seal joint, zygapophyseal, Z-joint; these joints are the interconnecting joints joining vertebral bodies one to another.

Asymptomatic

The opposite of symptomatic; refer-ring to absence or resolution of symptoms.

Atrophy

Wasting away. When referring to muscle, it generally implies reduc-tion or absence of enervation (nerve supply) secondary to nerve damage. May also, however, occur with re-duction in blood supply as well as enforced rest as might occur with casting a limb for an extended pe-riod.

Biochemistry

Refers to those aspects of chemical reactions that occur in living tissues. Example: cellular metabolism

Biofeedback

A psychotherapeutic technique used to assist patients in understanding the mechanism of self-regulation of the body. By giving feedback to the patient relating to changes in autonomic nervous system functions such as blood pressure, heart rate, skin temperature, sweat gland activity and muscle tension, patients become aware of their ability to consciously control physiological activities including muscle tension. This technique has become an effective adjunct in the treatment of pain syndromes such as migraine, muscular contraction headaches and other chronic pain syndromes.

Biomechanics

The mechanical movement of living tissues, generally referring to joint mechanics as influenced by the surrounding soft tissues defined by ligaments and muscles.

Botox (botulinium toxin A)

Has a wide range of therapeutic uses. When injected into muscle, Botox blocks the neurotransmitter acetylcholine from transmitting nerve impulses, therefore stopping the muscle from contracting. When abnormal muscle spasms are identified in whiplash-associated disorders, selective injection of Botox into these muscles can assist in relieving muscle spasm.

Cervical collar

An orthopedic support device, also called a neck brace. Useful in acute cervical trauma, the cervical collar provides relief by supporting the neck and head relieving the muscles from their duty of keeping the head upright. A towel wrapped around the neck and secured with tape may provide the same support.

Cervical spine

The specific seven vertebral bodies that comprise the top portion of the spine, beginning immediately under the skull and coursing downward to the torso at the upper shoulder level. These vertebral bodies are the most likely injured during the whiplash-associated injury.

Cervicogenic headache

Headache patterns that are thought to emanate from structures in the upper neck. Also referred to as muscular contraction headaches or tension headaches, they generally are thought to represent injury and irritation to the spinal nerves originating in the upper cervical spine.

Chiropractic

Chiropractic is a health care profession that focuses on diagnosis, treatment and prevention of mechanical disorders of the musculoskeletal system, with special emphasis on the spine. This health science is based on the hypothesis that these disorders affect general health via the nervous system. Chiropractors are extensively trained in manual therapy techniques that include both mobilization and manipulation.

Chronic pain disorders

Pain disorders that remain unresolved for a period greater than three months. Such pain syndromes often represent physiological and biochemical changes to the nerves themselves, which may result in sustained nerve malfunction contributing to the ongoing pain syndrome.

Craniosacral therapy

A manual therapy modality used by physical therapists, massage therapists, naturopaths, chiropractors and osteopaths for the treatment of dysfunctional movement patterns. Considered a complementary or alternative medicine technique, craniosacral therapy may be helpful in selected subjects in relieving neck pain associated with whiplash-associated disorders.

Diathermy

Three forms in wide use by physical therapists: shortwave, ultrasound and microwave. All are designed to direct heat to the subcutaneous tissues in the treatment of deep muscle and joint pain. Deep heat causes a temperature rise from the conversion of energy into heat as it penetrates the tissues of the body where the energy is applied. Energy sources include (1) high-frequency currents (shortwave diathermy), (2) electromagnetic radiation (microwaves), and (3) ultrasound (high-frequency sound).

Disc

The intervertebral discs are fibrocartilaginous cushions serving as the spine's shock absorbing system. Composed of an outer rind called the annulus fibrosus and an inner jelly-type substance called a nucleus pulposus, their content is predominantly water composed. During the whiplash injury the annulus fibrosus can be injured resulting in herniation of the nucleus pulposa, with contact and irritation of the exiting spinal nerve.

Dry needling intramuscular stimulation (IMS) A needling technique used in the treatment of chronic myofascial pain syndromes. Involves the repetitive insertion of acupuncture-type needles into muscular areas where muscle bundles are identified as shortened or contracted, or at points were muscles meet nerves. Developed by Dr. Chan Gunn, a Canadian pain specialist, this technique has been adopted as an efficacious pain therapy in selected cases throughout the world, for chronic, unremitting pain.

Generally practiced by physiotherapists and physicians trained in Dr. Gunn's institutes.

Dysfunction / dysfunctional   An abnormality, failure or malfunction of an anatomical structure resulting in its inability to function in a normal fashion. In relationship to spinal biomechanics, dysfunction results in loss of range of motion with change in muscular tone and development of pain syndromes.

Edema / swelling   Edema (American English) or oedema (British English) refers to the increase in fluid buildup between cells often as a response to injury. Referred to as interstitial fluid (fluid between cells); when associated with injury, edema is often accompanied by heat and swelling as might be noted after spraining an ankle.

Electrophysiology   Nerve cell electrical processing ability. Electrophysiology is the study of the electrical properties of biological cells and tissues. In the study of nerves, we are concerned with the propulsion of electrical impulses representing instructions to the muscles to produce contraction. In the opposite direction, electrical impulses from the periphery represent information being directed back to the spinal cord and brain relating to sensation, pain and proprioception.

Electrotherapy	Electrotherapy may be used in a variety of stimulation types, protocols and uses in the treatment of myofascial complaints. Neuromuscular Electrical Stimulation (NMES), transcutaneous electrical nerve stimulation (TENS), and interferential currents are all commonly used treatments in the relaxation of muscle spasm and rehabilitation. Peer-reviewed research articles have suggested that medical properties of the various electrotherapies may be useful modalities in treatment of these complaints. A subset of electrotherapy, electromagnetic therapy with the application of magnets to affected tissue is more controversial in terms of medical evidence. Therapy is normally provided by the use of electrode pads placed on the skin. Therapeutic effects are thought to occur from the increase in blood flow, stimulation of muscles and triggering of the release of endorphins, hormones that act as natural pain killers.
Epidural injections	A way to deliver pain medications into an area near the spinal cord called the epidural space. This epidural space contains the spinal nerves and allows medication directed into this space to come in di-

rect contact with these nerves. Generally epidurals are used to deliver steroid medications to inflamed spinal nerves.

Ethyl chloride stretch and spray A myofascial therapeutic regimen involving the spraying of a vapocoolant (ethyl chloride) over the skin of the painful muscular area, followed by stretching techniques to relieve trigger points and underlying muscular spasm. In theory, the external cooling stimulates receptors in the skin, allowing a break in the positive feedback loop affecting muscle spasm and accompanying pain syndrome. Initially recognized in the 1940s as beneficial, this technique was popularized by Travell and Simon.

Facet joint See apophyseal joint

Fascia Fascia is a soft tissue component that permeates the entire human body. Surrounding muscles, bones, organs, and nerves and blood vessels, fascia represents an uninterrupted three-dimensional web of tissue that supports our architectural frame. Depending on the amount of the elastin and collagen comprising fascial structures, the fascial component may describe a delicate web or a substantial supporting band overlying a muscle group. In soft tissue injuries, this extensive framework may be significantly disrupted and become a major contributor to accompanying pain syndromes.

Foramen	A Latin term referring to a tunnel-like passage formed either by bone or fascia, generally to allow an artery or nerve to pass peripherally. The foramen may also serve as protection.
Functional techniques	A manual therapy practiced by physiotherapists and osteopaths for correction of dysfunctional movement patterns identified in joint mechanics.
Heat	The application of heat (thermotherapy) is a time honored tradition in the treatment of injured tissues. It is particularly helpful for muscles that are in spasm. It works by increasing oxygenated blood flow and increases the extensibility of the tissues. Moist heat tends to penetrate deeper than dry heat. Care should be taken not to have direct contact of the heat with the underlying skin. Treatment duration is generally 20 minutes.
Herniated disc	Injury to an intervertebral disc resulting in extrusion of an innermost component of the disc (nucleus pulposa) and compression and irritation of the adjacent exiting spinal nerve; see disc.

Histopathology

Microscopic cellular abnormalities. Histopathology—from the Greek *histos* (tissue) and *pathos* (suffering)—refers to the microscopic examination of tissue in order to study the manifestations of disease. Damaged tissues show evidence of change of cellular structure implying inability to function normally.

Hyperextension

The process of bending backwards as opposed to the process of bending forwards (flexion).

Ice

A traditional therapy (cryotherapy) used in treatment of conditions of acute inflammation. Acute inflammation describes conditions where there is an influx of blood and interstitial fluid (fluid between the cells). Application of cold causes contraction of blood vessels and reduces this process. It should be applied for approximately 20 minutes, taking care not to damage the skin by having the ice directly contact the skin. This therapy is normally applied within the first 72 hours following injury.

Inflammation

The body's response to injury; generally refers to an influx of blood cells and body fluids in an attempt to effect a healing process; often accompanied by heat and swelling.

	Pain is generally an accompaniment of this process due to the distention of the tissues.
Intervertebral disc	See disc.
Kinesiology	Kinesiology, also known as human kinetics, is the science of human movement. This discipline focuses on how the body functions and moves. A therapeutic kinesiological approach applies scientific and evidence-based medical principles towards the analysis, preservation and enhancement of human movement in all settings. In rehabilitative settings, exercises are designed to restore function of posture, strength and movement.
Ligaments /Tendons	Ligaments are short bands of tough, fibrous connective tissue generally composed of long, stringy collagen fibers. Their purpose is to provide mechanical support for joints to control physiological range of motion. Tendons are composed of the same dense connective tissue but unlike ligaments, which connect bone to bone, tendons connect muscle to bone, such as the Achilles tendon, which connects the strong calf muscle to the ankle.
Malalignment	In relation to spinal biomechanics, refers to spinal alignment altered from neutral plane position. This may be secondary to muscular spasm more pronounced on one side

than the other or a dysfunctional movement problem affecting one or more of the facet joints.

Manipulation/Mobilization Describes various manual therapy techniques practiced by therapists for the purpose of restoring normal spinal biomechanics. These therapeutic techniques are generally instituted having determined evidence of dysfunctional movement patterns affecting adjacent vertebral body biomechanics.

McKenzie therapies A system of manual therapy involving applied mechanical forces by a trained therapist, with active patient involvement. Treatment algorithms were originally developed by physiotherapist Robin McKenzie and training programs for McKenzie therapists are found worldwide. Used extensively in the treatment of whiplash-associated injuries, they are effective modalities in the treatment of dysfunctional movement patterns.

Mild Traumatic Brain Injury (MTBI) A variety of physical, cognitive and emotional symptoms that follow minor head trauma, also known as concussion. Although commonly associated only with the transient loss of brain function, symptoms may persist and result in permanent damage. MTBI may be experienced in whiplash injuries, even without loss of consciousness

	or contact of the injured person's head with vehicle, other passengers, or cargo.
Motor function	Relative to nerves, refers to the specific nerves whose primary function relates to transmitting electrical impulses to the muscle to produce contraction, thereby creating motor function. Other nerve fibers may relate specifically to sensory function.
Muscle energy technique	An osteopathic manual therapy used to treat dysfunctional movement patterns of facet biocechanics, to regain normal range of motion in identified joint structures. Treatment requires patient participation and therapies generally include exercise programming, which the patient is able to perform between treatment sessions without the aid of the therapist.
Muscle relaxants	A class of drugs that effects skeletal muscle function and decreases muscle tone. Used to alleviate pain symptoms resulting from muscle spasm.
Muscular contraction headache	Describes headaches with a primary cause relating to increased tension of muscles at the base of the skull and upper neck. The increased tension in the muscle is thought to compress the exiting spinal nerves

in this area resulting in the headache experienced. Also called tension headache or cephalgia.

Myofascial pain syndrome A medical term used to describe regional sensitivity and pain affecting muscle and fascia. Often accompanied by trigger points, these conditions tend to be chronic in nature and often occur as a result of trauma. Many types of therapy are used in management; response to treatment is often described as idiosyncratic, meaning what works in one person may not work in the next.

Neural sheath A sleeve which encloses a group of nerve fibers. Individual nerve fibers enclosed within the neural sheath or sleeve may provide either sensory or motor function.

Neuropathic pain medications A group of drugs known for their anticonvulsant properties, used as antiepileptic drugs to control seizures. These drugs have also been found to assist in the relief of neuropathic pain syndromes. Gabapentin and pregabalin are examples of this class of drugs.

Neuropathic pain syndromes A significant pain syndrome resulting from damage or dysfunction of nerves resulting in hypersensitization of pain sensation. Pain syndromes tend to be out of proportion to the tissue injury and are often accompanied by burning, tingling and other symptoms, termed *paresthesias,* indicative of nerve dysfunction.

Neutral plane alignment   In reference to vertebral body spinal biomechanics, indicates normal position of vertebral bodies in relationship of one to its adjacent neighbor. Denotes absence of any dysfunctional movement pattern.

Nucleus pulposa   See disc.

Occipital nerves   Spinal nerves emanating from the upper cervical spine, which provide motor and sensory function to muscles and soft tissues of the upper neck and scalp; dysfunction of these nerves are thought to be instrumental in headache patterns experienced in whiplash injuries.

Osteoarthritis   The natural degenerative process affecting joints, associated with age. The predominant feature of osteoarthritis involves the loss of cartilage on joint surfaces. Most people will have osteoarthritis by the fourth decade but it may start earlier in those joints subjected to trauma.

Osteoporosis   A condition resulting in loss of bone mineral density, generally associated with aging, resulting in alteration of bony micro-architecture predisposing individuals to fractures with minimal trauma. Osteoporosis is most common in women after menopause but may develop in men as well. Certain medications or hormonal problems may predispose individuals to osteoporosis.

Palliative therapy   A recognition that a specific condition or disease process is unlikely to resolve spontaneously or even with treatment. Goals of therapy at this point relate to focus on best efforts at pain relief and improving function and quality of life.

Postmortem   After death. Postmortem examinations are those studies carried out in autopsies.

Post Traumatic Stress Disorder (PTSD)   A severe and ongoing anxiety disorder developing after exposure to one or more terrifying events that threatened or may have caused significant physical harm. This condition displays biochemical changes in the brain and body that differ from other psychiatric disorders such as major depression.

PRFN (percutaneous radio-frequency neurotomy)   When the facet joint has been identified as a specific pain generator in individual whiplash-associated disorders, percutaneous radio-frequency neurotomy (PRFN) can be used to temporarily interrupt the nerve supply going to this joint, thereby altering the pain sensation

	experienced. If successful, the treatment may have to be repeated at intervals to provide ongoing relief.
Prognosis	A medical term denoting a doctor's opinion as to how a patient's disease or condition will progress and whether or not there is a chance for recovery.
Proprioception	Describes the neurological function whereby we sense the relative position of neighboring parts of our body. For example, with our eyes shut we are able to determine whether or not our hand is open or closed.
Referral pain	Pain that refers along the course of the nerve even though the point of injury may be somewhat distanced from where the pain is felt. A typical example is *sciatica*, in which the problem is a pinched nerve in the back although the pain is felt in the leg. Referred pain may also be experienced in the arm and hand even though the pain source is a pinched nerve in the neck.
Scoliosis	An abnormal side bending or lateral rotation of the spine when viewed from back to front. This may exist from birth or be acquired during teenage years. Although exact causes are unknown, there appears to be some genetic predisposition. Severe cases may require medical intervention. To be differentiated

from *acquired scoliosis*, a correctable cause. See acquired scoliosis.

Shortwave diathermy	See diathermy.
Shoulder girdle	A composite term referring to the upper torso skeletal structures—*scapula (wing bone or shoulder blade), clavicle (collarbone) and spine*—and supporting soft tissue structures—*muscles, fascia and ligaments*—that serve as the foundation for the movement of the upper extremities.
Sniff position	An abnormal postural position whereby the head and neck are held in a forward position as might be illustrated by someone moving about the kitchen trying to find the source of a bad odor.
Soft tissue injury	A generalized term to indicate injuries that result in disruption of the architectural structure of the supporting muscles, ligaments and fascia. As opposed to skeletal injuries resulting in fractures, these injuries are considered a diagnoses of exclusion, after ruling out other possible causes, inasmuch as no specific medical test can prove or disprove their existence.
Spinal cord	The major track of nervous tissue that begins at the base of the brain and runs through the protected spinal column down to the base of the spine. At each level of the spine,

the spinal cord gives off individual spinal nerve roots, which course to different parts of the body, providing motor and sensory function.

Spinal nerve root blocks   Injections of medication onto or near nerves. In the treatment of whiplash, these injections normally include anesthetics and steroids. Generally undertaken with the use of fluoroscopy, a type of real-time imaging allowing accurate placement of the needle tip to the site of the nerve for delivery of the medication.

Spinal nerves   Exiting nerves from spinal cord. Between each vertebral body and its adjacent neighbor, a specific spinal nerve exits to provide sensory and motor function to a specified anatomical area.

Splinting phenomenon   A term used to describe the body's attempt to protect injuries by increasing muscular tension on all surrounding sides to prevent movement. A typical example would be spasms of muscles surrounding a skeletal fracture to prevent movement across the fracture line. Both back and neck injuries are significantly marked by splinting phenomena.

Steroids

A class of drugs used to treat many different conditions. Steroids used in the treatment of inflammation are generally in injectable form and are directed at sites for their local effect, reducing regional inflammation. Particular areas of interest in the treatment of whiplash relate to the facet joints as well as the spinal nerves at the point where they exit through the foramen.

Stress reduction

Muscle tension syndromes are markedly affected by increases in stress. Techniques designed to improve the subject's ability to recognize and manage stress have significant impact on overall level of comfort. Many different stress reduction techniques are recognized to achieve this effect. They may include distraction activities varying from playing a musical instrument or participating in athletic activities, to meditation and other consciousness-affecting techniques.

Subluxation

A term used by chiropractors in reference to dysfunctional movement and malalignment of vertebral body spinal segments. Manual therapy techniques are used to correct these dysfunctional movement patterns.

TENS (transcutaneous electrical nerve stimulation)

See electrotherapy.

APPENDIX A: GLOSSARY

Therapeutic modalities A broad term in reference to the many types of therapy used in the treatment of soft tissue injuries. May include massage, physiotherapy, manipulation, mobilization, soft tissue manual therapies, acupuncture, injection therapies, etc.

Trigger points Trigger points are bands of palpable nodules in muscular bellies. Also described as contraction knots, they are very tender to palpation and may be responsible for localized as well as referred pain. Trigger points often accompany myofascial pain syndromes seen in whiplash-associated disorders.

Trigger-point injections A therapy widely practiced in management of myofascial pain syndromes. Trigger points are knots or bands identified in spastic muscles. Local anesthetics, corticosteroids, saline or sterile water are all descriptions of injection fluids used in the treatment of trigger points. There is considerable debate as to whether one injection fluid is more efficacious than another; the physical disruption of the trigger point by the injection fluid itself may be contributing to the treatment's effectiveness.

Ultrasound therapy   A form of diathermy which uses high-frequency sound waves as a heat source in treatment of inflamed joints and muscles. Administered by a physical therapist, ultrasound produces heat, which penetrates deeply into the tissues to which it is directed. The rationale behind ultrasound therapy is that the production of heat is thought to stimulate healing by improving circulation and speeding metabolism. As in all heat-generating therapies, there is the potential for burns. It is not recommended for use near pacemakers, over the abdomens of pregnant women or over the skull, eyes or reproductive organs.

Whiplash-associated disorder (WAD) Describes the various symptoms that accompany injuries experienced in whiplash.

Reading Notes:

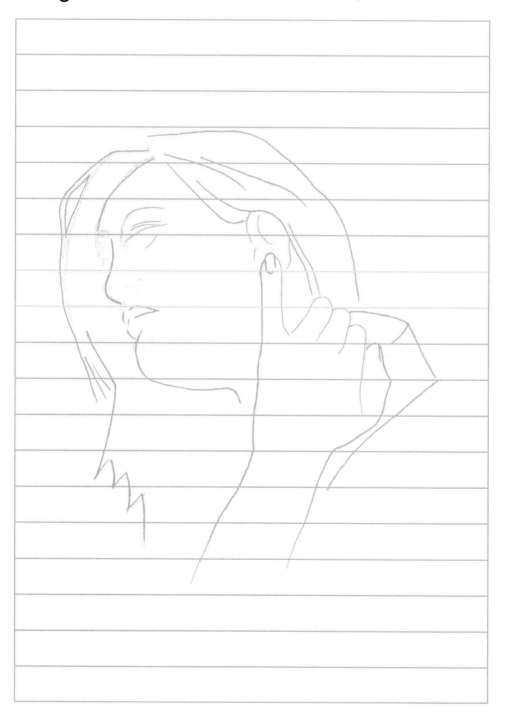

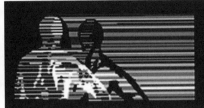

Chronic Back Pain Clinic
www.ChronicBackPainClinic.com
604-531-0444

Patient Name: _____

Date of Injury: _____

Time of Injury: _____

Town or City and Street where Crash Occurred: _____

What was the estimated damage to your vehicle? _____

Did the police come to the accident scene and make a report?

☐ Yes   ☐ No

Is an attorney representing you? Name / Address / Phone:

AUTO ACCIDENT DESCRIPTION:
Describe How the Crash Happened:

Collision description:

Check All That Apply to You: In the accident you were the:

☐ single car crash   ☐ driver
☐ rear end crash   ☐ front passenger
☐ head-on crash   ☐ rear passenger
☐ Two vehicle crash
☐ side crash (T-boned)
☐ hit guard rail / tree
☐ more than three vehicles
☐ rollover
☐ ran off road

MVA Questionaire 1

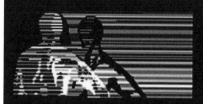

Chronic Back Pain Clinic

www.ChronicBackPainClinic.com
604-531-0444

Describe the vehicle you were in
Model, Year and Make:

Describe the other vehicle:
Model, Year and Make:

☐ Sub Compact Car
☐ Compact Car
☐ Mid-Sized Car
☐ Full-Sized Car
☐ Pickup Truck
☐ Larger Than 1 Ton Vehicle

☐ Sub Compact Car
☐ Compact Car
☐ Mid-Sized Car
☐ Full-Sized Car
☐ Pickup Truck
☐ Larger Than 1 Ton Vehicle

Estimated crash speeds

Estimate how fast your vehicle was moving at time of crash: _____
Estimate how fast the other vehicle was moving at time of crash: _____

At the time of impact **YOUR** vehicle was:

At the time of impact the **OTHER** vehicle was:

☐ slowing down
☐ stopped
☐ gaining speed
☐ moving at steady speed

☐ slowing down
☐ stopped
☐ gaining speed
☐ moving at steady speed

During and after the crash, Your Vehicle

☐ kept going straight, not hitting anything
☐ kept going straight, hitting car in front
☐ was hit by another vehicle
☐ spun around, not hitting anything
☐ spun around, hitting another car
☐ spun around, hitting object other than car

Describe yourself during the crash
(check only the areas that apply to you)

☐ you were unaware of the impending crash.
☐ You were aware of the impending crash and relaxed before the collision
☐ you were aware of the impending crash and braced yourself
☐ your body, torso, and head were facing straight ahead
☐ you had your head and /or torso turned at the time of collision -- turned to left -- turned to right (circle one)
☐ you are intoxicated (alcohol or drugs) at the time of crash
☐ you are wearing a seatbelt
☐ you are holding onto the steering will at the time of impact

MVA Questionaire 2

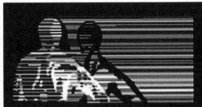

Indicate if your body hit something or was hit by any of the following:
(please draw lines and match the left side to the right side)

head	windshield
face	steering wheel
shoulder	side door
neck	dashboard
chest	car frame
hip	another occupant
knee	seat
foot	seat belt

Check if any of the following vehicle parts broke, bent, or were damaged in your car:

☐ windshield
☐ steering wheel
☐ dash
☐ seat frame
☐ side /rear window
☐ mirror
☐ knee bolster
☐ other --
☐ other --

Yes / No questions:

Yes No

☐ ☐ Did any of the front or side structures, such as the side door, dashboard, or floor board of your car, dent inward during the crash?

☐ ☐ Did the side door touch your body during the crash?
☐ ☐ Was your hand (s) on the steering wheel or dash during the crash?

☐ ☐ Did your body slide under the seatbelt?
☐ ☐ Was the door (s) of your vehicle damaged to the point where you could not open the door?

Rear end collision only:
Answer this section only if you are hit from the rear.

Does your vehicle have:

☐ movable head restraints
☐ fixed, non-movable head restraints
☐ no head restraints

Please indicate how your head restraint was positioned at the time of the crash.a

☐ at the top of the back of your head
☐ midway height of the back to your head
☐ lower height at the back of your head
☐ located at the level of your neck
☐ located at the level of your shoulder blades (upper back) below neck

Estimate the distance between the back of your head and the front of the head restraint.

_____ inches

MVA Questionaire 3

135

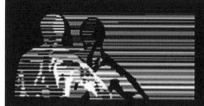

Chronic Back Pain Clinic
www.ChronicBackPainClinic.com
604-531-0444

Yes No
☐ ☐ Did you go to the emergency department after the accident?
    Name of Hospital: _____
    Date: _____
    Time: _____

Yes No
☐ ☐ Did you go to the emergency department in an ambulance?
☐ ☐ Did you or another person drive you to the emergency department?

    ☐ myself   ☐ another person

Yes No
☐ ☐ Were you hospitalized or observed in the emergency department overnight?
☐ ☐ Did the emergency room doctor take x-rays? Check which x-rays were taken:

    ☐ skull
    ☐ neck
    ☐ low back
    ☐ arm or leg

Yes No
☐ ☐ Did the emergency room doctor give you pain medications?
☐ ☐ Did the emergency room doctor give you muscle relaxants?
☐ ☐ Did you have any abrasions, cuts or lacerations?
☐ ☐ Did you require any stitches for cuts?

When did you first notice any pain after injury?

☐ Immediately
☐ _____ hours after injury
☐ _____ days after injury

If you did not see a doctor for the first time within the first week, indicate why (check all that apply)

☐ no pain was noticed
☐ work /home schedule conflicts
☐ no appointment time available
☐ no transportation

If you did not see a doctor for the first time within the first month after injury, indicate why (check all that apply)

☐ no pain was noticed
☐ work / home schedule conflicts
☐ no appointment time available
☐ no transportation
☐ I thought pain would go away
☐ I self treated with over-the-counter drugs
☐ I took hot showers, used ice, heat

Yes No
☐ ☐ Have you been unable to work since injury?
☐ ☐ Have you had to change your work duties since your injury?

Please list dates off work: _____ to _____

MVA Questionaire 4

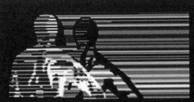

Chronic Back Pain Clinic
www.ChronicBackPainClinic.com
604-531-0444

HEAD INJURY QUESTIONNAIRE (fill only if head injured in accident)

Check What Your Head Hit or What Hit Your Head:

- [ ] No head injury
- [ ] Windshield
- [ ] Dashboard
- [ ] Other passenger
- [ ] Steering wheel
- [ ] Sidecar window
- [ ] Mirror
- [ ] Other _____

What part of your head was hit?

- [ ] Front
- [ ] Left side
- [ ] Top
- [ ] Back
- [ ] Right Side
- [ ] Other:_____

Please circle appropriate answer

Yes No

Yes	No	
		Did you lose consciousness or blackout for any time (seconds or minutes) after your head injury? How long?_____
		Have you lost in the memory of events before the head injury?
		Have you lost any memory or has your memory been different since the head injury?
		Did you have a lump or bruise after the head injury? Where?
		Have you had any head injuries in your past (include childhood)?
		Have you had any x-rays taken?
		Have you had a CAT scan or MRI scan taken of your head?

HAVE YOU EXPERIENCED ANY OF THE FOLLOWING SINCE YOUR NECK OR HEAD INJURY?

- [ ] headaches
- [ ] loss of coordination
- [ ] reduced drive / motivation
- [ ] poor memory
- [ ] difficulty finishing tasks
- [ ] sleep disorders
- [ ] abnormal levels of anxiety
- [ ] reduced tolerance to alcohol
- [ ] more assertive
- [ ] forgetful
- [ ] anger outbursts
- [ ] depression
- [ ] fatigue
- [ ] absence of ability to anticipate
- [ ] inflexibility
- [ ] impaired sexual function
- [ ] language difficulty
- [ ] impaired judgment
- [ ] need daytimer or reminder to remember home and / or work activity's
- [ ] blurry vision
- [ ] loss of balance

- [ ] difficulty handling multiple tasks
- [ ] dizziness / lightheadedness
- [ ] irritability
- [ ] personality change
- [ ] hand tremors
- [ ] ringing in the ears
- [ ] less diplomatic than normal
- [ ] mood swings
- [ ] reduced attention span
- [ ] blackouts
- [ ] indifference to other people
- [ ] more shallow relationships
- [ ] difficulty with solving problems
- [ ] less mental stamina
- [ ] performance inconsistencies
- [ ] verbal learning problems
- [ ] slower reaction times

MVA Questionaire 5

137

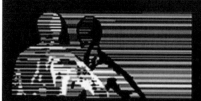

Chronic Back Pain Clinic

www.ChronicBackPainClinic.com

604-531-0444

If you have experienced any of the symptoms below, place a "X" in the box in front of the symptom and a checkmark in each of the boxes of the four categories to describe it. (may include more than one.)

		Felt Right After Injury	Felt 24-48 Hours Later	Have Symptoms Now	Had Similar Symptoms 1 to 3 Months Before This Injury
Example: X	*Headache*	X	X	X	

Headache					
Dizziness					
Tinnitus (Ear Ringing)					
Blurry Vision					
Memory Problems					
Poor Concentration					
Irritability					
Balance Problems					
Loss of Coordination					
Sensitivity to Sound					
Sensitivity to Light					
Fatigue					
Anxiety					
Pain / Difficulty Swallowing					
Jaw Pain					
Neck Pain / Soreness					
Neck Stiffness					
Shoulder Pain / Stiffness					
Arm Pain / Tingling / Numbness					
Wrist / Hand / Finger Pain / Numbness					
Weakness in Arms / Legs					
Upper / Mid Back Pain					
Chest Wall Pain (Rib)					
Low Back Pain / Soreness					
Hip Pain					
Leg Pain					
Leg Numbness / Tingling					
Pain Shoots down Legs					
Knee Pain					
Ankle / Foot Pain					
Other					

MVA Questionaire 6

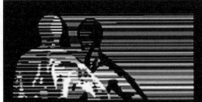

Chronic Back Pain Clinic

www.ChronicBackPainClinic.com

604-531-0444

Have you experienced any of the following since your motor vehicle accident?

☐ headaches	☐ difficulty handling multiple tasks
☐ loss of coordination	☐ dizziness / lightheadedness
☐ reduced drive / motivation	☐ irritability
☐ poor memory	☐ personality change
☐ difficulty finishing tasks	☐ hand tremors
☐ sleep disorders	☐ ringing in the ears
☐ abnormal levels of anxiety	☐ less diplomatic than normal
☐ reduced tolerance to alcohol	☐ mood swings
☐ More assertive	☐ reduced attention span
☐ forgetful	☐ blackouts
☐ anger outbursts	☐ indifference to other people
☐ depression	☐ more shallow relationships
☐ fatigue	☐ difficulty with solving problems
☐ absence of ability to anticipate	☐ less mental stamina
☐ inflexibility	☐ performance inconsistencies
☐ impaired sexual function	☐ verbal learning problems
☐ language difficulty	☐ slower reaction times
☐ impaired judgment	
☐ need daytimer or reminder to remember home and / or work activities	
☐ blurry vision	
☐ loss of balance	

MVA Questionaire 7

139

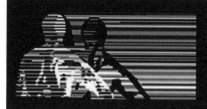

Chronic Back Pain Clinic
www.ChronicBackPainClinic.com
604-531-0444

Prior Treatment Questions:

LIST THERAPISTS, TESTS AND TREATMENT SINCE INJURY:

Start with the first doctor, chiropractor or therapist / office / hospital you saw after injury and check all that apply:

1

Name of / Doctor / Therapist / Center:

_____

Address: _____ Date:_____

Type of Therapy: (eg. physio, massage, chiro.)

_____

How many visits? _____

Indicate what was done:

- Exam -- Consultation
- X-Ray of Neck
- X-Ray of Low Back
- Other X-Rays
- MRI / CAT Scan
- Other Diagnostic Test
- Rehabilitation
- Physical Therapy
- Exercise Recommended
- Medications Prescribed
- Neck Collar
- Spinal Manipulation / Adjustments
- Muscle Massage / Physiotherapy
- Low Back Brace
- Heat Packs Cold / Ice Packs
- Ultrasound
- Other

Indicate results of treatment and therapy:

- helped but came back when I stopped treatment
- helped a bit and I kept my improvement
- didn't help at all
- made it worse

2

Name of / Doctor / Therapist / Center:

_____

Address: _____ Date:_____

Type of Therapy: (eg. physio, massage, chiro.)

_____

How many visits? _____

Indicate what was done:

- Exam -- Consultation
- X-Ray of Neck
- X-Ray of Low Back
- Other X-Rays
- MRI / CAT Scan
- Other Diagnostic Test
- Rehabilitation
- Physical Therapy
- Exercise Recommended
- Medications Prescribed
- Neck Collar
- Spinal Manipulation / Adjustments
- Muscle Massage / Physiotherapy
- Low Back Brace
- Heat Packs Cold / Ice Packs
- Ultrasound
- Other

Indicate results of treatment and therapy:

- helped but came back when I stopped treatment
- helped a bit and I kept my improvement
- didn't help at all
- made it worse

MVA Questionaire 8

140

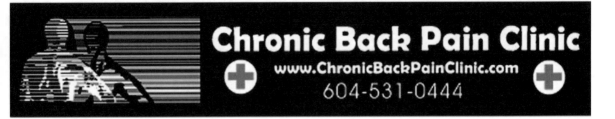

Prior Treatment Questions:

LIST THERAPISTS, TESTS AND TREATMENT SINCE INJURY:

Start with the first doctor, chiropractor or therapist / office / hospital you saw after injury and check all that apply:

3	4

Name of / Doctor / Therapist / Center:

_____

Address: _____ Date:_____

Type of Therapy: (eg. physio, massage, chiro.)

_____

How many visits? _____

Indicate what was done:

☐ Exam -- Consultation
☐ X-Ray of Neck
☐ X-Ray of Low Back
☐ Other X-Rays
☐ MRI / CAT Scan
☐ Other Diagnostic Test
☐ Rehabilitation
☐ Physical Therapy
☐ Exercise Recommended
☐ Medications Prescribed
☐ Neck Collar
☐ Spinal Manipulation / Adjustments
☐ Muscle Massage / Physiotherapy
☐ Low Back Brace
☐ Heat Packs Cold / Ice Packs
☐ Ultrasound
☐ Other

Indicate results of treatment and therapy:

☐ helped but came back when I stopped treatment
☐ helped a bit and I kept my improvement
☐ didn't help at all
☐ made it worse

Name of / Doctor / Therapist / Center:

_____

Address: _____ Date:_____

Type of Therapy: (eg. physio, massage, chiro.)

_____

How many visits? _____

Indicate what was done:

☐ Exam -- Consultation
☐ X-Ray of Neck
☐ X-Ray of Low Back
☐ Other X-Rays
☐ MRI / CAT Scan
☐ Other Diagnostic Test
☐ Rehabilitation
☐ Physical Therapy
☐ Exercise Recommended
☐ Medications Prescribed
☐ Neck Collar
☐ Spinal Manipulation / Adjustments
☐ Muscle Massage / Physiotherapy
☐ Low Back Brace
☐ Heat Packs Cold / Ice Packs
☐ Ultrasound
☐ Other

Indicate results of treatment and therapy:

☐ helped but came back when I stopped treatment
☐ helped a bit and I kept my improvement
☐ didn't help at all
☐ made it worse

MVA Questionaire 9

141

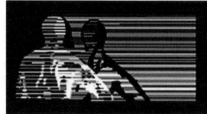

Chronic Back Pain Clinic
www.ChronicBackPainClinic.com
604-531-0444

Prior Treatment Questions:

LIST THERAPISTS, TESTS AND TREATMENT SINCE INJURY:

Start with the first doctor, chiropractor or therapist / office / hospital you saw after injury and check all that apply:

5	6

Name of / Doctor / Therapist / Center:

_____

Address: _____ Date:_____

Type of Therapy: (eg. physio, massage, chiro.)

_____

How many visits? _____

Indicate what was done:

- ☐ Exam -- Consultation
- ☐ X-Ray of Neck
- ☐ X-Ray of Low Back
- ☐ Other X-Rays
- ☐ MRI / CAT Scan
- ☐ Other Diagnostic Test
- ☐ Rehabilitation
- ☐ Physical Therapy
- ☐ Exercise Recommended
- ☐ Medications Prescribed
- ☐ Neck Collar
- ☐ Spinal Manipulation / Adjustments
- ☐ Muscle Massage / Physiotherapy
- ☐ Low Back Brace
- ☐ Heat Packs Cold / Ice Packs
- ☐ Ultrasound
- ☐ Other

Indicate results of treatment and therapy:

- ☐ helped but came back when I stopped treatment
- ☐ helped a bit and I kept my improvement
- ☐ didn't help at all
- ☐ made it worse

Name of / Doctor / Therapist / Center:

_____

Address: _____ Date:_____

Type of Therapy: (eg. physio, massage, chiro.)

_____

How many visits? _____

Indicate what was done:

- ☐ Exam -- Consultation
- ☐ X-Ray of Neck
- ☐ X-Ray of Low Back
- ☐ Other X-Rays
- ☐ MRI / CAT Scan
- ☐ Other Diagnostic Test
- ☐ Rehabilitation
- ☐ Physical Therapy
- ☐ Exercise Recommended
- ☐ Medications Prescribed
- ☐ Neck Collar
- ☐ Spinal Manipulation / Adjustments
- ☐ Muscle Massage / Physiotherapy
- ☐ Low Back Brace
- ☐ Heat Packs Cold / Ice Packs
- ☐ Ultrasound
- ☐ Other

Indicate results of treatment and therapy:

- ☐ helped but came back when I stopped treatment
- ☐ helped a bit and I kept my improvement
- ☐ didn't help at all
- ☐ made it worse

MVA Questionaire 10

APPENDIX C:
CARE PROVIDERS AND CREDENTIALS

Acupuncturist

One who is trained in the ancient Chinese therapy of acupuncture. Acupuncture involves the insertion and manipulation of fine needles into specific points on the body, with the aim of relieving pain and achieving a wide variety of therapeutic purposes. The body of scientific evidence supporting acupuncture is active and growing suggesting that acupuncture may be particularly helpful in treatment of musculoskeletal conditions. There is general agreement that acupuncture is safe when administered by well-trained practitioners using sterile needles. Most acupuncture points are geographically related to arteries and nerves and may be used by other practitioners as a geographical map for injection therapy.

Anesthesiologist

An anesthesiologist is a medical doctor who has undertaken additional postgraduate training in anesthesia. Although anesthesiologists are most recognized as the doctors that put you to sleep before surgery, some anesthesiologists specialize in pain management therapies. These therapies involve injection therapies in an attempt to alter pain response.

143

APPENDIX C: CARE PROVIDERS AND CREDENTIALS

Chiropractor

Chiropractors, also known as doctors of chiropractic or chiropractic physicians, in many jurisdictions are primary-contact health care practitioners who emphasize the conservative management of the neuro-musculoskeletal system without the use of medicines or surgery. Chiropractors place special emphasis on treatment of spine conditions. They are extensively trained in manual therapy techniques that include both mobilization and manipulation.

Interventional pain physician Describes a large group of variously trained physicians including neuroradiologists specializing in interventional pain therapies. See neuroradiologist.

Kinesiologist

A kinesiologist is one who, after obtaining a university degree in kinesiology, practices the discipline of kinesiology. Kinesiology, also known as *human kinetics*, is the science of human movement. This discipline focuses on how the body functions and moves. A kinesiological approach applies scientific and evidence-based medical principles towards the analysis, preservation and enhancement of human movement in all settings. In rehabilitative settings, exercises are designed to restore function of posture, strength and movement.

Massage therapist

One who is trained in the therapeutic modality of massage. Massage therapy is probably the oldest of physical therapies, dating back to pre-biblical times. With over 80 known different massage modalities, techniques are designed to be applied with hands, fingers, elbows, forearms and feet, with the intention of acting upon or manipulating soft tissue structures. Although there are many therapeutic benefits relating to massage therapy, in musculoskeletal injuries, techniques are employed to restore normal myofascial function. Training programs vary from jurisdiction to jurisdiction but generally involve studies in anatomy and physiology, kinesiology and instruction in different soft tissue techniques.

Naturopath

One who practices naturopathic medicine. Naturopathic medicine is an alternative or complementary medicine which emphasizes the body's intrinsic ability to heal and maintain itself. Naturopaths prefer to use natural remedies such as herbs and foods rather than drugs. Some naturopaths have additional training in physical medicine to include manual therapy, exercise therapy and various injection therapies including prolotherapy.

APPENDIX C: CARE PROVIDERS AND CREDENTIALS

Neuroradiologist

Neuroradiologists practice a subspecialty of radiology focusing on the diagnosis and characterization of abnormalities of the central and peripheral nervous system, spine, head and neck. Neuroradiologists use the primary imaging modalities including plain radiography, CAT scans, MRI and ultrasound. Some neuroradiologists specialize further in interventional neuroradiology. Using image-guided spine intervention, injection therapies can be directed specifically to intraspinal spaces, spinal nerves or facet joints.

Osteopathic physician

Osteopathic physicians have training similar to medical doctors and generally carry out all the functions that medical doctors do in general practice. In addition, osteopaths emphasize the role of the musculoskeletal system in health and disease. Osteopaths are trained in and use a wide range of manual and physical treatment interventions in the treatment of musculoskeletal problems including back and neck pain.

Physiotherapist

One who practices physiotherapy or physical therapy. Physical therapy describes a wide spectrum of rehabilitative services with many subspecialties including cardiopulmonary, geriatrics, neurological, orthopedic and pediatric services. The span of education ranges from undergraduate degrees to masters and doctoral qualifications. In relationship to whiplash-associated disorders, physiotherapists vary widely in training but therapeutic modalities may include mobilization/manipulation, therapeutic exercise, neuromuscular reeducation, hot and cold packs, electrical stimulation, ultrasound and other therapies used to expedite recovery in an orthopedic setting.